D0139401

# STORIES OF RESILIENCE IN NURSING

Ideas about resilience and identity continue to be promoted, discussed and debated in nursing. This book uses narratives to explore these complex and important concepts, unsettling our certainties and opening up new perspectives on what they might mean and involve.

This engaging book recounts direct and vivid stories told by or about nurses. These vignettes discuss nursing's ideals without idealising them and show nursing work and the lives of nurses in all their complexity. They include contributions from mental health nurses, a former nurse, student nurses, a migrant nurse and a whistle-blowing nurse, among others. The book ends with chapter-by-chapter contextual material to promote reflection, discussion and further reading.

Written with nursing students preparing to transition to the workplace and professional status in mind, this thought-provoking book is also suitable for nurses and nurse academics interested in resilience and issues around professional identity.

**Michael Traynor** is Professor of Nursing Policy at Middlesex University, London, UK, where he works in the Centre for Critical Research in Nursing and Midwifery.

TOURO COLLEGE LIBRARY
*Kings Hwy*

WITHDRAW

WITHDRAWN

# STORIES OF RESILIENCE IN NURSING

Tales from the Frontline of Nursing

*Michael Traynor*

TOURO COLLEGE LIBRARY
*Kings Hwy*

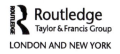 Routledge
Taylor & Francis Group

LONDON AND NEW YORK

3699

κH

First published 2020
by Routledge
2 Park Square, Milton Park, Abingdon, Oxon OX14 4RN

and by Routledge
52 Vanderbilt Avenue, New York, NY 10017

*Routledge is an imprint of the Taylor & Francis Group, an informa business*

© 2020 Michael Traynor

The right of Michael Traynor to be identified as author of this work has been asserted by him
in accordance with sections 77 and 78 of the Copyright, Designs and Patents Act 1988.

All rights reserved. No part of this book may be reprinted or reproduced or utilised
in any form or by any electronic, mechanical, or other means, now known or
hereafter invented, including photocopying and recording, or in any information
storage or retrieval system, without permission in writing from the publishers.

*Trademark notice*: Product or corporate names may be trademarks or registered trademarks,
and are used only for identification and explanation without intent to infringe.

*British Library Cataloguing-in-Publication Data*
A catalogue record for this book is available from the British Library

*Library of Congress Cataloging-in-Publication Data*
Names: Traynor, Michael, 1956– author.
Title: Stories of resilience in nursing : tales from the frontline
of nursing / Michael Traynor.
Description: Abingdon, Oxon ; New York, NY : Routledge, 2020. |
Includes bibliographical references and index.
Identifiers: LCCN 2019018425 | ISBN 9781138485129 (hbk : alk. paper) |
ISBN 9781138485136 (pbk : alk. paper) | ISBN 9781351050272 (ebk)
Subjects: | MESH: Resilience, Psychological | Nurse's Role |
Nursing Process | Personal Narrative
Classification: LCC RT41 | NLM WY 87 | DDC 610.73–dc23
LC record available at https://lccn.loc.gov/2019018425

ISBN: 978-1-138-48512-9 (hbk)
ISBN: 978-1-138-48513-6 (pbk)
ISBN: 978-1-351-05027-2 (ebk)

Typeset in Bembo
by Newgen Publishing UK

9/29/20

# CONTENTS

# FIGURES

# PART I

# 1

# LET ME TELL YOU ABOUT THIS BOOK

It has often been said that we learn through stories. We discover, or invent, who we are—heroine, observer or victim perhaps. In stories we surround ourselves with our group—it could be our fellow student nurses—and distance ourselves from the 'other'—managers, doctors, qualified nurses or patients perhaps. Stories are everywhere. This book will use stories to explore the transition from student or trainee to nurse, as well as aspects of being a nurse.

Since the mid 1990s, qualified nurses, health visitors, district nurses, mental health nurses, managers and midwives, as well as students and support workers, have told me their stories in focus groups and in one-to-one interviews. My early-career research was to do with probably the first major reorganisation of the National Health Service (NHS), involving the introduction of so-called market forces. A language and an ethos from the world of business started to be used by politicians about caring for patients. Some managers I interviewed were excited about this new world: one ambitious nurse executive enthusiastically showing me his new electronic organiser, a clunky precursor to today's smartphones. However, nearly all the nurses I interviewed were appalled. They told me that they did the real work and that managers were only interested in the finances of the organisation. In phrases that have reverberated ever since, they told me how little they thought managers cared about them and what they did. They told me stories of rushing through work with frightened elderly patients crying in their homes. Some years later, when 'evidence-based medicine' was being taken up across healthcare, nurses talked to me about how they were making clinical decisions. Their accounts were made up of vividly remembered first-person stories, sometimes of how a single nurse, the teller of the story, 'somehow' sensed that a patient was more seriously ill than their colleagues or doctors had realised—and was proved right. Shortly after this, nursing in the UK and elsewhere came in for bad press following revelations of poor and apparently cruel care dished out by nurses in Stafford in the UK, as well as in other parts of the country. The profession as a whole was poised on the edge of a serious fall from grace. At that time, student nurses studying in both mental health and adult branches of nursing told me how shocked they were by the poor patient care that they saw and how they believed that a caring nature was something that an individual nurse either had or did not have. Many told stories of conflict with and among qualified nurses. I began to notice that some students appeared to understand that systemic problems, such as poor staffing levels, unstable organisational structures and badly supported ward managers, had a big influence on how nurses behaved and how patients were cared for. Others appeared to blame poor nursing on bad nurses. It seemed to me that the first group of students had taken a slight distance from the distress of what they had witnessed in a way that the second group had not. They did this, I think, by acknowledging that there was a story behind the behaviour and events that they encountered.

But what unites these distinct research projects undertaken over 25 years is the way that groups of nurses naturally turn not to text books or theoretical concepts but to storytelling when they want to explore ideas about their work and their own identity. And it is stories that are foregrounded in this collection.

Ten chapters of this book are stories based on data I have collected from my research studies, other interviews, informal conversations as well as meetings arranged specifically for this book with student nurses, healthcare trainees, qualified nurses and a few individuals who have left the profession. The research studies had their own particular questions to answer but here I have let the words spoken take centre stage. The stories have been assembled along with some supporting material into these ten separate narratives. Pseudonyms have been used throughout and I have gone to great lengths to anonymise the tellers, sometimes changing the context of their original stories. So if you have spoken with me, you may find echoes of your words in these pages but not where you might expect them. Taken together, the chapters of this book set out their own story. The beginning tells stories of people thinking about becoming nurses or who are in training, the middle shows us the transition across the border between student and qualified nurse, the end presents stories of people who have been in the profession for many years or who have decided to move or leave. The intention behind this book is that the experience of reading these stories and then discussing them in the classroom or with colleagues will change the way you might understand what it is to be a nurse.

The other strand that unites these stories is that they all have something to say about resilience in its different forms. Resilience is the subject of many texts and articles and it was the topic of my last book. I was and am sceptical about the way that the idea of resilience has been used in nursing. Too often it is seen as an alternative to change, an alternative to challenging dysfunctional and exploitative working situations—situations that may well compromise patient safety. Nurse writers who promote resilience among nurses often fail to distinguish between the trauma intrinsic to the work itself—dealing with sickness and death—and the organisational and political forces that sometimes feel like they are designed to make effective nursing as difficult as possible. Sometimes the narrators in this book talk overtly about resilience in the various ways they understand it, and sometimes it is never explicitly referred to. In Chapter 3 I will say a little more about resilience for those readers who are not familiar with discussion around it or who have not read the previous book.

## Nurses under pressure

Taken together with health visitors and midwives, nurses are the largest professional group employed within the UK's NHS today, making up 55% of the workforce (NHS Digital 2016). It is a similar story in most countries' health systems. With the UK government relentlessly implementing cost control across the welfare sector and 70% of hospital spending being on staff, nursing work is clearly in the frontline for pressure. The nurse-to-population ratio in the

UK is 8.2 per 1000 population (2014 figures), below the OECD[1] average of 8.9 per 1000 and representing a fall from its 2011 level (Charlesworth and Lafond 2017). This ratio is lower in the UK than Canada, Australia, the USA, New Zealand and the Scandinavian countries. The National Audit Office (2016) claims that the supply of clinical staff for the NHS in England is insufficient for the demand. It estimates a workforce shortfall of around 50,000 NHS staff, including 27,980 nurses. The House of Commons Committee of Public Accounts (2016) claims that this is a result of fewer nurses being trained, with the Department of Health cutting training places by 3,400 in 2012/13 from the 2008/09 level. The number of nurses in training has reflected the rises and falls in funding to the NHS as a whole and varies a great deal from year to year (Charlesworth and Lafond 2017).

So it is easy to see that many nurses work in situations that are likely to thwart their best efforts at delivering safe and high-quality care. Professional aspirations and ideals can only be maintained in such an environment with extraordinary effort and perhaps a degree of unremitting commitment that no employer has the right to expect from their workers, or indeed that is healthy and sustainable. Training, of course, also takes place in this context. That it works as well as it usually does is a tribute to the dedication, imagination and flexibility of students and mentors alike. That it is often, too often perhaps, unsatisfactory is entirely predictable. The need for nurses and those in training to understand the causes of their dissatisfaction is urgent, along with the need for action to influence and change.

## How to use this book

This book can be used as a teaching aid for nurse education. It makes an ideal companion to final year modules that deal with professional identity or the transition to qualification. It can be used in the classroom to start discussion about nursing work and nursing identity. Each chapter/narrative deals with different issues and can form the basis of one session, or two can be compared. The stories show nursing work and the lives of the individuals and groups who tell the stories or feature in them in their complexity, so any 'lessons' drawn are unlikely to be simple ones but they will, I hope, be both profound and useful. Each chapter is supplemented by material that provides suggestions and questions for tutors and students to open up each narrative.

But I think the stories have the ability to stand on their own and to have an effect on the reader without the intervention of either myself or others. Because of this, I have separated the teaching material I mentioned above largely into a chapter at the back of the book. There you will find sections that correspond to each narrative. There are also pointers to further background material. I separated the book in this way so that those who simply want to enjoy or be challenged by the stories and their emotional and other overtones can do so without the distraction of overtly didactic interruptions.

Finally, I have sourced some images for many of the chapters, some provided by the tellers of the stories and some from elsewhere.

I end this introduction with a quotation from Arthur Frank, whose ideas I will return to in the next chapter. It is taken from his book about storytelling and analysis, *Letting Stories Breathe*. I place it here because I think it makes a good description of the stories in this book.

---

1 The Organisation for Economic Co-operation and Development (OECD) is an intergovernmental economic organisation with 35 member countries, founded in 1961 to stimulate economic progress and world trade.

… [good] stories do not present themselves as simple models for action. They do not direct action directly but conduct it by indirection. Characters in good stories do not exemplify what anyone anywhere must do: they are doing what *they* have to do, where and when they find themselves.

*Frank 2010, p. 160; my emphasis*

## On a personal level

On a personal level, this book is an attempt to deal with some unfinished business: the mystery and trauma of my own history and involvement with nursing and, at one remove, another history and involvement with National Socialism, in that part of my family grew up in Nazi Germany, subsequently emigrated and failed to engage with the horrors and reality of how the Nazi project implicated the whole nation. I keep returning to what has been referred to as *Trümmerliteratur* and *Trümmerfilm*, creative work focussing on the immediate post-war ruin and trauma in Germany. One (of many and highly recommended) works looking back on this period is *Europa* (1991), an early film by Danish director Lars Von Trier.

Though, of course, a satisfying and important profession, for me—and some readers of this book—nursing will never be far away from trauma.

# 2

# A TALE TOLD BY A NURSE...

In this chapter I set the scene for the stories that follow by talking about the study of narrative. I draw on the work of well-known teller of tales Arthur Frank among others. The chapter summarises a history of storytelling from aboriginal myths, through ancient Greek drama, religious stories, medieval mystery plays, Shakespeare (...full of sound and fury) and modern drama, to reality television and YouTube. It presents a summary of research and reflection on professional socialisation and its relationship to resilience.

## Narrative, story and narrative research

'This book will change the way you think and feel about your life'. The claim appears on the front cover of my edition of *Zen and the Art of Motorcycle Maintenance,* a novel by Robert Pirsig (1983), first published in 1974, shortly before I was born. That cover makes quite a claim. Though I am not sure that thinking and feeling are unentwined, the idea, I think, is that stories have a mysterious power to do something to us through the enjoyment of encountering them, even when the stories themselves might be unsettling or a little heavy-handed, as Pirsig's book turned out to be.

Despite the decision to put the stories centre stage in this book, I want to frame them by talking about what stories are and how stories have been used in the nursing and healthcare professions. However, I want to tell you at the start that this book is not a textbook about narrative research. Think of this book as fiction, a collection of short stories. The only difference is that the stories here are true stories that happened and continue to happen.

## What are stories?

To understand human life many look to the stories that individuals and groups circulate among themselves—the stories that are told and believed in. Aboriginal groups are well known for sharing stories about their origins and the origins of the land and creatures around them (see http://dreamtime.net.au/). Their stories, for example about the birth of the Emu, are often enigmatic and obey a logic that most contemporary Western readers or listeners do not share. They are considered to be a way of maintaining culture and identity in an oral society and of teaching skills and values to new generations.

More familiar to Europeans, though equally enigmatic, are ancient Greek myths and the scriptural stories of the Abrahamic religions.[1] These stories also feature accounts of origins—of the world, god(s) and humans. They include a supernatural realm of origin and influence on the affairs of women and men. Apart from communal entertainment, these stories, particularly those associated with what we now tend to separate out from the rest of life and think of as 'religion', appear to have served the purpose of maintaining strong group identity in the context of nomadic encounters with other tribes. These stories provide explicit teaching about acceptable and unacceptable behaviour in the form of laws originating from supernatural sources. The stories also form the basis of subsequent interpretations and reinterpretations as sanctioned teachers and scholars look for enduring principles that can guide the lives of those who believe in them.

The messages and morals of Greek drama tend today to be debated by literature scholars and psychoanalysts, rather than theologians and religious leaders. At the centres of these stories are kings and other powerful figures who, often with the noblest of motives, struggle against the inexorable powers of fate. They captivate us as audiences by evoking pity and horror, at Oedipus[2] stabbing out his own eyes after realising he has killed his father and had sex with his mother, to take just one example. Such dramatic figures have become known, unsurprisingly, as 'tragic heroes', often brought to terrible ruin by the playing out of some 'flaw' in their character, a flaw that can simultaneously be seen as an admirable quality, wanting to know the truth in Oedipus' case.

One aspect of public storytelling across Europe in medieval times[3] took the form of 'mystery' or, later, morality tales. Performed in the vernacular rather than Latin—the language of church services—and with plenty of spectacle, music and detailed stage directions, the plays generally presented religious allegory. As these plays were sanctioned by the church and performed from the back of a cart in the street, their purpose was clearly public religious education. Morality plays featured personifications of various moral attributes, such as Perseverance, Pity or Good-Deeds, and a protagonist who represented humanity as a whole—'Everyman' as he is called in one well-known play from the period—rather than what we think of today as an 'individual' character. We have to wait until Shakespeare (1564–1616) to find stories that combine the externalised personification of evil—the witches in Macbeth for example—with the 'internal' struggles of conscience of Macbeth himself or, famously, of Hamlet. We have learned to recognise in their soliloquies the processes of thought that are just like our own: 'why am I not doing the thing I know I should be doing? Why am I drawn to do the thing I know will have terrible consequences?'

While ancient myths featured gods and Shakespeare's dramas focused on the lives of kings, queens and warriors, dramatic stories in the modern age have come to hold up the lives of

---

1 Judaism, Christianity and Islam: all considered to originate from the monotheistic practice of the historical figure of Abraham.

2 Oedipus was a king in Greek mythology, ruling over the city of Thebes. He was the son of King Laius and Queen Jocasta. Unknowingly, he married his mother and had four children with her, among them Antigone (https://en.wikipedia.org/wiki/Oedipus). The play *Oedipus Rex* (Oedipus the King) was written in approximately 430 BC by the Athenian playwright Sophocles.

3 Approximately from the 5th to 14th centuries in Europe.

ordinary people for examination, sympathy and sometimes admiration. *Death of a Salesman* by American playwright Arthur Miller, first performed in 1949, features an ordinary 'everyman', the travelling salesman Willy Loman. The play shows the effect of the 'American dream' on the life and family of this failing and ultimately deluded individual. An 'ordinary hero' like Willy Loman is said to be easier to identify with than Athena or Perseverance.[4] In film, British New Wave cinema underlined a move toward a dramatic focus on the reality of ordinary, often neglected, working-class lives. This movement lasted from the late 1950s to the early-to-mid 1960s and included, by most counts, ten highly influential films on unromantic, uncomfortable topics, often looked at critically. By this point in this short history of Western storytelling, we are a world away from the tales of kings, gods and heroes. Both Miller and the filmmakers associated with the British New Wave were politically motivated but their concerns also reflect a strongly individualising move in most Western societies. In fact there is a kind of contemporary inversion at work, with the ordinary individual elevated to the status of hero or god in reality television, true-life media stories and YouTube video making. In today's highly individualised societies, more people than ever before are publicly telling their own stories, whether about an illness, a trauma, an opinion or a product.

## Stories are everywhere

Today, stories are as influential as ever. They are at work even when we do not realise it. In his book *Letting Stories Breathe*, Arthur Frank (2010) provides many instances of contemporary stories and their effects, for example the stories about the founder of an American insurance company that are told and retold by employees and that seem to give them a sense of corporate duty and belonging. The company with the right corporate story seems to keep its staff better than others in the area.

In my last book about resilience I included a story told by a resilience researcher that seems to create a paradigm case of resilience:

> Sara was the youngest of four children raised in a dysfunctional family environment. Her father was an alcoholic and her mother was physically and verbally abusive. After years of fighting and yelling, Sara's parents ended up in a bitter and protracted divorce. Sara's needs were a low priority in the family chaos. Sara was a chubby baby, who turned into a chubby kid, who turned to food for most of her comfort. Despite her expanding waistline and often being the subject of cruel teasing, Sara knew she was smart as a whip and could always rely on her sense of humor to get her out of a tough situation. Sara had one best friend who lived down the street; her name was Jenny. Sara and Jenny shared everything: they conspired to grow up and have fantastic lives. Sara was going to become a pediatrician and help sick children, get married, and have a perfect house with three kids. Meanwhile, Sara's family continued to spiral down. They had stopped going to church, dropped out of the social functions they used to attend, and lost contact with family friends. Sara often found herself home alone or left at school until early evening, forgotten by her parents. Nonetheless, she did not bother to complain, tried to stay out of her parents' way, and generally took everything in stride. She dreamed of the

---

4 The development of the 'everyman hero' across popular culture can be seen as making the idea of the resilient individual, who succeeds in the face of adversity, a coherent and attractive prospect for research and policy.

day she would be off to college and medical school, working hard to become a doctor. Sara grew up in that environment until she was 17. She did go off to college with a full academic scholarship. Once there she joined Jenny Craig, lost 60 pounds during her freshman year, and went on to enjoy social events and make new friends. She is a happy, practicing pediatrician today.

*Earvolino-Ramirez 2007* [5]

Although this model story foregrounds Sara and her thriving against the odds, it is the background elements, easily, perhaps casually, chosen because they are so readily available, that interest me. These are the positive social values by which health, success and resilience are measured: friendship, family life, opportunity, education, hard work, professional success, being slim and being 'happy'. Perhaps this is the real meaning and message of the story: the story could perhaps be titled 'What is the good life in America today?' The story also tells us that dreams can be achieved and that the achievement of dreams merits a story being told so that others can be encouraged also to have a dream. Perhaps the story even provides a rough framework for the kind of dream that we can dream. So the story in a way shapes even what feel like our most personal dreams.[6]

## Narrative research

I promised that this book would not be a textbook about research methods, but I want to include some paragraphs here that summarise one approach to the study of narrative because it will allow you to read the stories here in a more sophisticated way.

Narrative research includes a number of approaches to social science research that examine the written or spoken words of individuals in order to investigate a research question. Narrative analysts understand the stories of individuals as sources of data and tend to focus on chronology and other elements of structure within stories to enable and support analysis. These approaches often focus on the lives of individuals as told through their own stories. Like other labels applied to research methods however, the term narrative analysis covers a wide variety of techniques, interests, purposes and fundamental starting points with regard to beliefs about truth and human identity. From my perspective, some of these approaches miss the point of stories altogether. That is because, I believe, they approach stories from the orientation of fundamentally wanting to use them to answer a research question and to come up with a coherent account of the topic under study and an analysis that can be set out under discrete themes. The more interesting approaches allow stories to 'breathe' to use Arthur Frank's word

---

5 I tried unsuccessfully to contact the author of the paper that this passage is taken from. I wanted to ask whether this was a 'real' story of apparent resilience or a fictitious illustration of what some people mean when they talk about 'resilience'. (She calls it a model case.) I can't help noticing that the protagonist of the story, Sara, has a best friend called Jenny and then later in her life joins the weight-loss organisation Jenny Craig. The same author has also published on strategies and barriers for managing weight. The 60 pounds that Sara lost in a year is equivalent to 27 kilograms, or a little over 4 stone.

6 It has become a common statement in psychology, pop and otherwise, that the type of story we chose to tell about our lives in some way 'creates our personality' (McAdams and Manczak 2015). This type of claim assumes, I think, that there is someone—a homunculus, a miniature man—sitting at the controls inside the individual and making decisions about things, including how to tell the story of their life. I invite you to think about the opposite and perhaps counter-intuitive idea that it is the stories already existing, circulating and having unseen influence that tell the person.

from the title of his book on the topic (Frank 2010). Stories we tell and hear, enjoy and live by can be full of nuance and contradiction. The identities of the storyteller that they create, or that they call us to become, can be incoherent and fractured. Their attempt at generating a unified identity can 'fail'. If we are too keen to approach stories only as a resource that can help us come up with answers to social science questions, we can miss out on the appreciation and even enjoyment of these features. We can also miss out on realising that however much a teller protests and believes that they are telling their 'own' individual story, 'anyone's story presupposes both other stories and the recognition of other people. People's stories are their own, but people exist only in dialogical relationships, and stories also express a relation' (Frank 2010, p. 192). One example of this, which you will find in nearly all of the stories in this book, is the story participated in by nurses that nurses nurse out of caring and a desire to make a difference to the lives of their patients.

Narrative analysts set out various characteristics that they suggest need to be present in order to detect the presence of a story, for example time and place, human agency or categories of narrator. Sociolinguist William Labov proposed an influential schema, the elements of which he claims are present in a complete oral narrative: an abstract, an orientation, a complicating action, an evaluation, a resolution and a coda or signal that the story is complete (Labov 1972).[7] Some analysts do their work to get a more accurate understanding of the structure of narrative, or language, or dialect and sound change, as does Labov. Others study personal narrative to understand the interaction of social and historical processes with the realm of the personal, as does feminist sociologist Katherine Riessman (1993).

## Psychoanalysis and stories

Psychoanalysts also draw on stories to develop theories that go far beyond the drive to understand the structure of narrative. The 'founding father' of the discipline Sigmund Freud (1856–1939) interpreted existing myths to explain puzzling characteristics of the human psyche. Freud looked to the story of Oedipus that I mentioned above as he developed the idea of the 'Oedipus complex'. This complex describes, he believed, normal stages in a child's psychic development. The theory was developed from Freud's analysis, published in 1909, of 'Little Hans', a five-year-old boy who had a phobic fear of horses (Freud 1990). To put it simply Freud suggested that all small boys make their mother their first object of developing sexual desire. They unconsciously wish to usurp their father's place as her lover and harbour a jealous desire to exclude their father. According to Freud, most boys successfully negotiate this process and emerge with a new separation from their mother, which is essential for healthy adult life. Freud discussed a similar, though far from identical, process for girls, which some have called the Electra complex, also a reference to Greek mythology.

Freud also developed his own 'myths', as in his account of the 'primal horde' (Freud 2001). He recounted this speculative story of the early history of humans in order to account for the enduring presence and power of religions. He claimed that, in primitive societies, people lived

---

7 To give a little more detail (from various sources): the abstract announces what the story is going to be about; the orientation sets the scene and provides further context, often in terms of who? what? when?; the complicating action refers to the core of the story, the problem, perhaps; the resolution provides narrative closure, a solution to the complicating action; the evaluation makes the point of the story clearer; and the coda tells us that the story is finished and we are back in the real world.

in 'hordes' arranged around a single dominant male. This male had sole claim to the females in the group. Freud argues that the other males in the group murder this dominant authority figure out of jealousy. However, they are subsequently tormented by great guilt. This guilt passes down unconsciously through generations and the males begin to focus this sense of guilt on an animal, a 'totem', to whom they make sacrifices to atone for their unconscious sense of having committed an unspeakable crime. Over time the totem has been replaced by a more abstract 'God' figure to whom various sacrifices and devotions are still offered, along with the emergence of the telling concept of 'original sin' in the Christian religion (i.e. Adam and Eve's sin, whose 'guilt' all humanity unavoidably shares).

Most contemporary accounts of this theory and of Freud's use of the Oedipus myth end by saying that nobody today takes these speculations seriously. Nevertheless, they have reverberated in Western culture ever since he proposed them—nearly everyone has at least heard of the 'Oedipus complex'—and they have created a style of inquiry that many others have built on and developed in contemporarily sensitive ways. I mention them here because I want to emphasise the power and ubiquity of stories and storytelling, the stories that people live by, to use Arthur Frank's words again.

## How have stories been used in nursing?

Nursing, like any other line of work, including the selling of insurance policies mentioned above, surrounds itself with stories. In nursing, stories feature in a number of ways, both formal and informal.

### *As a formal part of nurse education*

Since at least the 1970s, nurse educators have used stories generated either by student nurses themselves or by patients (real or fabricated) as a learning resource and strategy. The rise of the use of storytelling was part of a reaction to what some educators felt was an over-emphasis on the scientific aspects of nurse education that characterised curricula on both sides of the Atlantic. Some educators have encouraged nurses to write stories about their own or their family's experiences of illness or healthcare. They argue that this can enable self-reflection and the development of empathy and understanding about the experience and perspective of others. This approach, however, tends to make certain assumptions that other more sophisticated understandings of stories and storytelling do not. For example, one recent teaching initiative in Scotland involved taking material from the website www.patientopinion. org.uk, a site where NHS patients can leave comments about their healthcare encounters. Student nurses were asked to analyse and discuss examples and write down what they had learned about how to practise (Tevendale and Armstrong 2015). Though apparently useful, the short patient and carer comments that were used are not stories in the sense that most analysts would understand them, even though they are presented in the context of traditional storytelling—they are simply comments, without the beginning, middle and end that are generally considered the minimum properties of a story. This approach, in the example above and in other places, tends to be highly formulaic—patient 'stories' feature compassion or a lack of it from nurses and the student nurses' response is to talk about having learned that compassion and good communication are vital parts of their practice.

A second kind of story used in nurse education is the historical tale, the story of the profession's founders—or founder depending on how you see it—and the development of the profession. There are few professions that still honour a single figure as their originator but the story of Florence Nightingale fits the bill as a story that might inspire nurses and student nurses today. Florence can play a number of characters. She was a reformer of the disreputable rag bag of occupations that went under the name of nursing in and prior to the early 19th century; she was a campaigner for a new line of work that respectable women could take up in a society where middle-class women were generally expected to organise and purify the home; she was brave, taking a group of personally trained nurses to the battle zone[8] of the Crimean peninsula, today part of the Russian Federation; she was a feminist who skilfully persuaded the politicians of the day to institute her ideas for nurse training; and she was even a scientist in the form of a collector and analyser of mortality data from the British military hospital in Turkey in the mid 1800s. She is easily recognisable too, once you get past the initial impression that all white Victorian women looked exactly like her and that all white Victorian men were identical with high foreheads and long beards. Other early heroic or influential nurses have more recently been brought onto the stage, for example Jamaican-born Mary Seacole, who also nursed wounded soldiers in the Crimea.

### As a way of understanding professional socialisation

The type of stories I mentioned above could be described as the profession's official stories, intentionally used by certain groups to build up the status of the profession as a whole, of certain aspects of professional ideology or of groups within nursing. The urge to tell stories, of course, exceeds any attempt to regulate it so unofficial and sometimes extremely uncomfortable stories circulate among nurses continually. But stories always serve some purpose and I would like to explore some of those purposes now.

Researchers and others have written a great deal about professional socialisation in nursing. For some examples see Melia (1987), Howkins and Ewens (1999), Mackintosh (2006), Brennan and McSherry (2007), Maben, Latter et al. (2007), and Allan, Traynor et al. (2016). One of my favourites is *Beyond Caring* by Daniel Chambliss (1996). He writes about how nurses deal with ethical dilemmas and relationships with doctors and managers, and particularly about how they respond to traumatic aspects of nursing work. Although his examples can more accurately be seen as examples of the use of humour—backstage, dark humour—rather than stories with the features we discussed earlier, taken together they can be seen as exploring the way that narratives can be used by nurses to 'routinise the traumatic' and loosen, to some extent, the tension caused by tragic or horrific events. This kind of literature shows us that learning to be a nurse involves learning to tell and recognise your place within the range of stories circulating among your colleagues and within the profession.

Other publicly available stories are very definitely examples of the 'backstage' humour that Chambliss gives examples of. The website Allnurses, the US-based 'leading social-networking site for nurses and nursing students', which has the slogan 'Knowledge empowers you', put out a call in 2002 for 'Your Most Gross, Yucky, Disgusting Nursing Horror Story'. At the time

---

8 The Crimean War lasted from 1853 to 1856.

of my visit, their invitation had received over 2000 responses (https://allnurses.com/what-is-your-most-gross-t17398/). Clearly, there is no shortage of nurses willing to share stories about highly taboo and often traumatic events. It is crucial, though, to consider the context of story-telling and story-listening if we are trying to understand the meaning of this activity. Whereas Chambliss and other researchers have gathered spontaneous or at least unsolicited stories from the workplace, perhaps during shifts or after the events that gave rise to the stories, it could be that the editors of the Allnurses website issued their invitation, at least in part, to drive traffic to their pages and improve advertising revenue. Nevertheless, such stories are part of nursing culture and many other social media spaces include a wider range of stories from practising nurses and students.

Finally, my own questions to nurses during research studies, for example into how nurses make clinical decisions, have often evoked highly dramatic stories as answers, as I mentioned in the previous chapter. The stories are often intended by their tellers to make points that would never be considered part of official nursing discourse—either this or their tellers are unaware of the underlying 'moral' of the story that they are telling. Examples include the story that I referred to in the last chapter about the patient who was more seriously ill than everyone believed except the teller, who knew this only by intuition, or stories that are underpinned by an assumption that 'doctor knows best' or that interprofessional working is fundamentally about hostility and getting the upper hand.

## How does storytelling relate to resilience?

It is quite common to hear an argument about storytelling and resilience that goes something like this: individuals can reflect on their lives and the adversity they have experienced. Through telling a story about these things, they give their lives a coherence and the adversity a meaning or at least a manageable form; in addition, from listening to these stories, others can learn that adversity can be overcome, as well as learning something about how this might be achieved, 'learning coping mechanisms from others who are more resilient' (Dyer and McGuinness 1996, cited in East, Jackson et al. 2010). In this argument, from nursing researchers, there is some cause and effect said to be at work—it is the act of telling the stories or listening to them that gives rise to resilience. Other writers only note an association. For example, Randall and colleagues asked twenty older people to answer a questionnaire that they believed would measure 'resilience' and then asked those who scored highest and lowest to tell stories about their lives. Not surprisingly, those who scored 'high' on resilience also told stories that featured characteristics that the researchers claimed showed a greater sense of agency and optimism, while those who scored 'low' tended to tell stories in which they were victims of events (Randall, Baldwin et al. 2015).

However, both types of research make some strongly individualistic assumptions. The first is the understanding of resilience as a psychological characteristic of individuals that can be assessed by asking those individuals a series of questions about themselves. Certain kinds of answers are given the label 'resilience', or sometimes 'hardiness'.[9] The second is that the

---

9 In Chapter 2 of my earlier book, *Critical Resilience for Nurses* (Traynor, 2017), I set out the case that the argument for the existence of resilience is circular. I also point out that today's common understanding of resilience has lost the environmental aspect that early resilience researchers believed was an essential aspect of explaining the differences between children who 'bounced back' from adversity and those who did not appear to.

stories people tell are 'their own'. I have summarised the arguments of some of those who have questioned this earlier in this chapter. While signifiers like 'nurse' or 'mother' will have different resonances for different individuals, people can only tell stories about themselves or anything else with material that is already widely accepted and recognisable as a story.

## Summary

I want to end this introduction by emphasising the point above about stories, and about identity in the process. There are other ways of approaching stories and I have mentioned some of these, but I find the following approach to be the most fertile, original and the least closed-down. 'My' story requires a 'you' to become possible. It is impossible to tell a story without an audience. Even a brief fantasy I develop about myself 'in my head' is for an audience—for a kind of 'other' that I habitually imagine witnessing my actions. So we do not develop stories alone—stories are not just 'our' stories. But not only are stories unavoidably 'dialogues' that require and presuppose an 'other' as the audience, the context for any story-telling goes far beyond teller and listener and is beyond the control and full understanding of both. What counts as a recognisable story and what counts as a recognisable individual is already established and circulating. In the same way that as infants we have to learn a language that is not 'ours' and has already existed long before our emergence, we can only tell a story within a set of norms that already exist. So in this sense, again, we have to question how far an individual's life story is 'theirs'.

Second, some believe that we are in some way not fully known—or knowable—to ourselves. How did I emerge or develop as a subject? I can never know because I would need to be already fully emerged and developed to witness this emergence to be able to give an account of it. In addition, I am not fully aware of the reasons for my perceptions, emotions and behaviour: when someone I know fails to greet me one day, why do I find myself feeling humiliated, guilty or, for a split-second, worthless? This unknowability is always a threat to the authority of the 'I' that I try to establish as the teller of my story. All I can do is tell story after story, each aiming at a kind of resolution of this problem and each, in a sense, failing. The advantage, in ethical terms, of understanding my failure to be coherent is that I may not demand absolute coherence and consistency from the stories of others. There is a view that good mental health involves being able to tell a coherent story of my life and that, if I am unable to do this, a number of eager therapists can help me to develop such a narrative. Of course we need to tell stories—it is unavoidable—but if we want someone to tell a coherent narrative of their life, it could be that we prefer the seamlessness of the story to the 'truth', the inevitable incoherence and contradiction, of the person. We might, reading this argument, feel the loss of a certain type of identity or self, but, according to this view, it is the loss of an identity that was never possible to begin with, a loss of what we never had (Butler 2001).

# 3

# RESILIENCE

## The story so far

At a recent event I attended on the theme of resilience, a member of the audience who had until recently worked as a district nurse in the UK spoke up. She told us that she had a caseload of over two hundred patients and that a total of nine of her patients had died during one single shift. Understandably traumatised by this experience, she told us how she asked her managers if there was any support available to her. The reply, we heard, was that she should do some resilience training. She went on to tell us how she subsequently discovered that a large number of colleagues in her team were taking anti-depressants to cope with the demands of their jobs. Soon after this she was diagnosed with post-traumatic stress disorder (PTSD)[1] and resigned.

The event, which was organised by the Royal College of Nursing (RCN) and held in London, was designed as a forum for discussion about different approaches to resilience. On the panel were an NHS nurse manager, two speakers from the *DNA of Care* project funded by NHS England, which collects audio-recorded stories from NHS staff, a worker from the RCN's counselling service, a PhD student whose research involved an investigation of resilience and myself. We were given a chance to set out our different approaches to resilience and to respond to questions from an audience of about 70.

My own interest in the topic started when I came across an article by radical economist Mark Neocleous. Neocleous suggests:

> 'Resilience' has in the last decade become one of the key political categories of our time. It falls easily from the mouths of politicians, a variety of state departments are funding research into it, urban planners are now obliged to take it into consideration, and academics are falling over themselves to conduct research on it.
>
> *Neocleous 2013, p. 3*

He also noted that the apparent usefulness of and need for resilience had become internalised by many individuals as they faced personal problems. Resilience is a term commonly heard

---

1 Rethink Mental Illness provides a list of some of what are considered to be symptoms of PTSD, as well as contact information for those who want help. See www.rethink.org/diagnosis-treatment/.

within healthcare organisations at the moment. Despite the very best intentions and the commitment of teams—both small and large—who provide resilience training, I think that the widespread promotion of resilience among healthcare workers, including nurses, ends up supporting the status quo and can leave staff who might be traumatised by organisational failures feeling personally responsible for those failures. I knew this was true in theory from my reading but testimony like that above shows us its operation in practice.

This chapter summarises material in my recent book to provide a background to the origins and development of resilience studies and the beginnings of a critique of the way that resilience has been used more recently. If you have read that book, you might want to skip to the next chapter. My argument, in my previous book and summarised at the event mentioned above, is that resilience today has become something of a fad that has been taken up by many groups, including some nurses and their managers, superficially without a proper understanding of where it came from or what has been left out on the way from the original concept. The notion of resilience has become increasingly individualised and popularly promoted as a set of behaviours that individuals can be taught and can make an effort to adopt.[2] Meanwhile, other disciplines have taken up the idea of resilience and tried to apply it to ecological and other systems in a strong departure from the individualised approach that appears to predominate in psychology, or at least in much of its public presentation.

## A very short history of resilience

How did the idea of resilience first gain popularity, at least in its current form? It was child psychologists and psychoanalysts working from the 1980s onwards who were puzzled by the observation that some children from challenging backgrounds appeared to conform to their problematic origins while others seemed to escape the negative and harmful influences and, apparently, thrive. Their work had its origins in the ideas of Sigmund Freud, widely considered to be the founder of the discipline of psychoanalysis, along with those who followed him and adapted (or challenged) his ideas. John Bowlby (1907–1990), for example, focused his work on children's early environmental experiences and argued that separation from a primary care giver could be associated with trauma at the time and social and emotional problems in adult life. In the many accounts of the origins of 'resilience' research, Bowlby is rarely mentioned. However, his theory of the benefits of attachment and interest in the effects of childhood trauma, coupled with his concern for direct observation of environmental events impinging on the child, set the context for later studies.[3] In the early days, writers such as James Anthony (1916–2014) talked about 'invulnerable' children (Anthony and Cohler 1987) but soon swapped this awkward description for the term resilient. Their model was that protective factors modified the impact of adversity on children, leading them to emerge in different ways. These protective factors could be operating at the neighbourhood, school, family or individual levels and operated in an interacting way. For Anthony, the most effective protective system was the infant's caregiver and their actions and precautions. Actions aimed at improving resilience tended to be community focused. In fact, early researchers in the field had the foresight to warn that the concept of

---

2 There are exceptions, of course, though not many. One of them is the work done by the Centre of Resilience for Social Justice at the University of Brighton in the UK. See www.brighton.ac.uk/crsj/index.aspx.

3 Michael Rutter, a later resilience researcher, thought that Bowlby overestimated the damage caused by infantile separation (Rutter 1985).

resilience could be misused by policy makers and politicians as an excuse to withdraw services and encourage the socially disadvantaged to simply shape up (Luthar and Cicchetti 2000).

However, as psychologists brought their characteristic methodology and techniques of individual measurement to bear within the field, an approach emerged in which the communal dimensions of investigations into resilience were dropped. Many researchers focused purely on the attempt to measure this mysterious resilience by means of the psychological questionnaires that we are all familiar with, one example being the Resilience Scale for Adults, a questionnaire with 37 questions designed to assess what the authors argue are the five dimensions of resilience: personal competence, social competence, family coherence, social support and personal structure (Friborg, Hjemdal et al. 2003). This particular scale was devised based largely on the lists of protective factors developed by some of the foremost resilience researchers over the previous 20 years and was created specifically to measure the presence of these attributes. This kind of work and investigation into so-called resilience has a different flavour to the more holistic investigations of environments and the individuals and groups within them. As one team of researchers has written:

> …many characteristics that appear to reside in the child are in fact continually shaped by interactions between the child and aspects of his or her environment…
>
> *Luthar and Cicchetti 2000, p. 864*

The following two standpoints articulated by different child resilience researchers show how an apparently subtle change in emphasis opens the way for a contemporary vision of resilience training as an alternative to social change:

> Some sources of adversity are preventable such as child maltreatment and it is far more effective to try to prevent these in the first place.
>
> *Masten and Obradović 2006*

> The primary concern of those working with children and adolescents at risk is the prevention of maltreatment and abuse, but given that this is not always possible, the promotion of resilience is even more valuable.
>
> *Williams and Hazell 2011, cited in Winders 2014, p. 7*

## Resilience research and nursing

The next problematic move comes with the adoption of resilience in nursing research. This is a growing field of work. Sometimes such work is done by researchers who are themselves nurses. Sometimes it is done by teams including psychologists and sometimes by nurses studying for PhDs with psychology supervision. Nurse researchers, in almost every piece of writing I have seen, understand resilience in purely individual—individualistic—terms. They give out questionnaires to nurses to measure their level of resilience, saying sometimes that this could help managers 'target' resilience training to those in most 'need' or at most 'risk'. None, to my knowledge, have attempted to assess whole organisations or units for resilience characteristics.[4]

---

4 It is not far-fetched to think that a resilient healthcare organisation would be one with built-in capacities and procedures that enable the maintenance of safe staffing levels even when a particular unit is short of staff due, for

In a review of resilience research in nursing, I identified what I consider to be a number of unhelpful characteristics:

1   Authors fail to differentiate between different types of 'adversity' that affect nurses. The first group of sources of adversity include exposure to and having to deal with patient suffering and death and the close relationships that may develop with these patients (e.g. Zander, Hutton et al. 2010, Dolan, Strodl et al. 2012). The second group of adversities, which is referred to often at great length, includes global nursing shortages and high turnover (e.g. Larrabee, Wu et al. 2010, p. 82), political change and under-resourcing of public healthcare (e.g. Koen, van Eeden et al. 2011), casualisation, staff shortages, bullying, abuse and violence (e.g. Jackson, Fau-Firtko et al. 2007). You could say that the first type of adversity is intrinsic to nursing work. The second can be seen as the direct effect of under-resourcing, political ideology, poor management, dysfunctional and insecure organisations, disempowered nurse managers, sexism or racism in the workplace, problems that all potentially result in understaffing and high turnover. All of these problems require action to address them, not the encouragement of nurses to 'thrive' on them.

2   There is a broad assumption that it is a free choice for a nurse to remain in the nursing workforce, that it provides evidence of a degree of resilience and that some of those who remain at the bedside apparently 'thrive' on the adversity they experience. There is also an assumption that a decision to leave nursing can be understood as succumbing to adversity, that is, a negative consequence, a sign of pathology. None of the work I have read entertains the possibility that nurses might remain in nursing because of a lack of local alternatives or that leaving the profession could be seen as a sign of strength and an appropriate response.

3   Many nurse researchers seem unaware of the history and debates within earlier resilience studies. Definitions of resilience in this literature show an over-reliance on other research written by nurses and perpetuate a partial understanding of the term. The nursing literature tends to draw on an 'internal' understanding of resilience as 'a positive personality characteristic' (Matos, Neushotz et al. 2010, p. 309).

4   Though 'adversity' is understood in organisational and workforce terms, there is little attempt to consider or measure this. The focus within this literature is almost entirely on individual personal responses and characteristics. Most studies are carried out in single sites so there is no opportunity to investigate whether any differences in resilience are associated with different ways of working (rather than differences in individuals). There is no conception or consideration of resilient systems in the nursing literature.

5   There is a tacit acknowledgement from the authors of powerlessness and that the workplace experienced by nurses is so dysfunctional that it is better to invest energy in devising personal approaches to coping than investigating or challenging the causes of the dysfunction. Promoting resilience among nurses is a way, according to many of the authors, of reducing turnover in the nursing workforce, with the promise that 'nurses can thrive at the bedside for "extended periods of time"' (Mealer, Jones et al. 2012, p. 297). According to some (presumably well-meaning) authors, the measurement of resilience

---

example, to sickness. To imagine, as some do, a resilient organisation as one where managers exhibit empathetic behaviour is the result of being unable to conceive of resilience as anything other than a personal characteristic.

can be used to identify those nurses with low resilience and target them for 'support' to help them to last longer. Some authors repeat in the introduction to their studies the unempowering mantra of resilience: 'you can't often choose what happens to you but you can choose how you react'. Paradoxically, at the same time as configuring the individual as one who bears responsibility to 'cope', they seem uninterested in talking to the individual to find out what adversity or protective factors mean to them with their unique history.

## Neoliberalism and responsibilisation

The widespread promotion of resilience is a child of its time. Its focus on individual responsibility and its neglect of consideration of structural factors resonates with a global political tendency toward neoliberalism.[5] Some commentators have used the term 'responsibilisation' to describe a tendency in the work of many Western governments today that takes the form of placing responsibility on individuals to avoid risk and make the most of opportunities to maximise their health, prosperity and independence (O'Malley 2009).[6] Nurses who go on resilience courses or who urge others to go are, it could be argued, playing into the hands of those who do not understand or perhaps value nursing work. And, what is worse, the phenomenon of resilience training perpetuates a contemporary mindset that promotes the 'naturalness' of the individual bearing responsibility for situations that are the making of others. The possibility of collective activity—resistance, challenge, systemic change—is simply not part of the horizon of possibilities.

## Is resilience any use?

Are we in danger of 'throwing the baby out with the bathwater', as I have often been asked? This is a good point to summarise my argument so far.

For the reasons that I mentioned above, the promotion of resilience has come to the fore in the UK and in nursing in today's NHS. Resilience has recent origins in research into child development and the relationship between the individual child and their environment. The complex concept of resilience has been simplified, first among the so-called 'psy' professions (such as psychology), many of which appear more interested in working at an individual level and less orientated to understanding social issues, by an almost exclusive focus

---

5 Narrowly defined, neoliberalism is an economic policy model that emphasises the value of free market competition. It is based on 19th century liberalism but it re-emerged in the 1970s in both the UK and US, at times of mounting public debt. However, it has wider resonances than the purely economic with its scepticism toward the usefulness of state interventions, such as the redistribution of wealth or provision of statewide social security and welfare. These props are seen as potentially demotivating for individuals. Neoliberal governments are often to be seen in conflict with public sector organisations and workers—the police, social workers, health workers and others. The proportion of government spending in these sectors tends to be reduced, sometimes sharply, during periods of administration by neoliberal governments.

6 Responsibilisation is 'the process whereby subjects are rendered individually responsible for a task which previously would have been the duty of another—usually a state agency—or would not have been recognized as a responsibility at all. The process is strongly associated with neoliberal political discourses, where it takes on the implication that the subject being responsibilized [!] has avoided this duty or the responsibility has been taken away from them in the welfare-state era and managed by an expert or government agency.'

on 'internal' characteristics and so-called skills. I suggest that resilience has been distorted or even exploited by those who realise that it can be co-opted into the 'responsibilisation' that some commentators believe characterises the kind of society we find ourselves in today. From this point of view it becomes part of a move, to put it crudely, to reduce investment in welfare. It has been taken up in nursing with the hope that it might ease the experience of nurses who work today under considerable, and some say unsustainable, pressures. However, much of the research and the interventions around resilience by nurses seem to neglect analysis of the causes of adversity for nurses and exhibit a sense of powerlessness and pessimism about dealing with the issues that make the apparent need for resilience so urgent in the first place. That is one reason why they tend to be so individually based. When a situation is intolerable, coping and resilience is not a good answer—attempting to change the situation or, if that fails, to leave it, seems a better, ultimately more healthy approach.

Many resilience studies and courses have been aimed at helping people to respond to, what we might call, the hand that life has dealt them: a terminal diagnosis, the death of loved ones. Resilience in the workplace is a very different matter. I pointed out earlier that resilience researchers in nursing have listed a number of causes of adversity. These all exist for specific reasons. Often they are the result of particular decisions or on-going strategies devised by particular groups. One example from the infamous Staffordshire trust involved saving on the organisation's staffing budget in order to be more likely to be successful in an application for Foundation Trust status, itself an incentive set up by a particular government for its own objectives and from its own political standpoint. But we have to ask who is likely to suffer the most from such policies? Perhaps those groups that make the least trouble. Many websites tell us that resilience is being 'able to roll with the punches'. As I said in my previous book, I think it is preferable to make sure you stop getting hit rather than to learn how to be able to last longer before you finally collapse.

There is another argument that nurses who have some personal resilience abilities are those who are more likely to be confident enough to act assertively, perhaps to challenge and change what is unacceptable in their environments and to protect themselves. I like this argument; however, I find no evidence or mention of this strategy in any of the research on nurses and resilience. It is more common to see resilience as a route to reducing an organisation's costs for recruitment and to reducing nursing turnover. Most child-development researchers have emphasised that resilience is as much a feature of the environment as of the child's characteristics and that interventions that do not include attention to the environment are unlikely to have lasting benefits.

The promotion of resilience covers over more complex and disturbing issues for the individual and organisations. You could say that this is one reason why it is so popular. The individual is left to deal with the issues themselves when so-called 'resilience' fails to help them. The organisation gets off the hook but never solves its basic problems.[7]

---

7 Allow me to predict the demise of resilience. While the use of the term resilience will become increasingly diffuse until it retains only the faintest meaning, it will be replaced by another urgent and attractive idea. Funding will be put into a new type of initiative, career planning for nursing associates perhaps. The number of those in influential positions who have critical tendencies and who express concern, for roughly the reasons I set out here, will grow. Many leaders are already uneasy about the potential for the promotion of resilience to blame 'victims'. And those with influence but with less critical tendencies will be eager to support, and be seen to support, the next initiative. They will be incentivised to do so.

## 'Critical resilience'

So, what is the alternative to this individualistic and politically submissive form of resilience? I put forward something to you that we could call 'critical resilience'.

Critical resilience is about understanding: understanding ourselves and our experiences in relation to our society—to take a phrase from feminist consciousness-raising groups (Chicago Women's Liberation Union 1970). The combination of becoming informed about the political and policy forces acting on day-to-day working life with frank, mutually supportive discussion can develop critical resilience. Neither is enough on its own. Reading a radical nursing blog on health policy or on the latest Nursing and Midwifery Council (NMC) initiative, if you can bear it, for example, is just the starting point for responding. And discussion without information can too easily turn into complaint, where the pleasure is not in the creative energy released by analysis and planning to do something but in simply repeating expressions of suffering. We all have experience of this.

Critique is a practice that demands a rigorous engagement with its object. It is also productive because it can lead to action. I suggested to nurses present at the event that I opened this chapter with, and I suggest to you as readers today, that we explore the possibility of setting up groups with fellow students or colleagues to develop informed critiques about aspects of working life. These could be place-based or asynchronous—a nice term to describe social media and web-based discussion forums that are present even for nurses who are isolated in whatever way. Becoming an active member of the RCN or other trade union is, clearly, a good first step.

Getting together and getting informed are the twin foundations for developing critical resilience.

## Oh no, not more 'C' words

I want to end this chapter by reiterating some thoughts from *Critical Resilience for Nurses* (Traynor 2017) about the differences between critique, criticism and complaint. I want to suggest that critique might open the way to compassion. Imagine a situation involving only two people—you and another nurse or manager for example. Imagine whatever you like about who they are and what they want of you. If you introduce a third term, you can escape this possibly claustrophobic situation (think of the infinite reflections you see when standing between two almost parallel mirrors). The third term here is a structure or theory, that is, a critique that you can apply from outside this dyad to try to make sense of the situation and the behaviour of that other nurse, other worker, or university tutor. Critique can free you from blaming individuals because structural explanations can give you an insight into some reasons (incentives and the threat of punishments for example) why another person might behave as they do. Here is a diagram to put this idea even more simply.

Nurse → critique → compassion

In this chapter I have set out a brief history of resilience, along with some critiques of research on resilience and, more importantly, of the way that this research has been attractive to governments and co-opted into a culture that is highly individualised. I have suggested that its take up in nursing research suffers the same individualising tendency. 'Resilience' seems to work as an enigmatic signifier, a kind of empty placeholder that different groups use in ways that are familiar to them or can further their interests. To move forward, I have introduced a concept that I think is more useful and called this 'critical resilience'. I have set out the difference between critique and other more familiar activities, like complaint. I have suggested that you explore the possibility of setting up groups with your fellow students or colleagues to develop informed critiques about aspects of working life.

With this in mind—resilience, its nuances and critiques—I now invite you to consider, experience and enjoy a number of stories that feature nurses in some relation to resilience of different kinds.

# PART II

# 4

# CAROL, THE NURSE WHO WENT ON STRIKE

In 2010 the UK government announced a cap of 1% on pay rises to public sector staff. The cap lasted until 2017. During these seven years, inflation continued at an average of 2.26%, hitting a maximum of 4.4% in 2011. In other words, nurses and their fellow public sector workers had their pay cut in real terms over this time.[1] According to the Royal College of Nursing, the 1% pay cap caused nurses' pay to fall by 14% in real terms during its existence, leaving them £3,000 a year worse off. The RCN also pointed out that low pay made it difficult to attract staff to fill the 40,000 nursing vacancies in England, with more nurses leaving than joining the register over that period.[2]

Nurses rarely go on strike. Though the nurses marched and protested on this issue, handing in a petition to the government to 'scrap the cap', the RCN did not call a strike. This is the story of a nurse who stood out and went on strike.

It was as recently as 1995 that the RCN revised its 'Rule 12' to allow strike action by nurses to be sanctioned on the proviso that such action was not 'detrimental to the wellbeing or interests of their patients or clients'. Before this change, the RCN's refusal to allow its members to strike was controversial. The RCN's council, its governing body, saw it a sign of its responsibility and professionalism. And it did hold a place on pay-determining bodies over the years. But among members of other unions and more militantly minded RCN members, the RCN's position was seen as a failure to live up to its trade union identity and as a lack of solidarity with other healthcare workers. There is, so far, no legal restriction on nurses taking strike action and the NMC Code does not prevent nurses and midwives from taking part in lawful industrial action; however, the RCN has never called for industrial action or a strike.

On 12th January 2016, junior doctors took part in a general strike across the NHS in England. This was the first time that doctors had taken such industrial action in 40 years. They went on to a series of five-day strikes (strictly speaking, strikes on five consecutive

---

1 For more details of UK inflation levels see www.statista.com/statistics/306648/inflation-rate-consumer-price-index-cpi-united-kingdom-uk-y-on-y/.

2 For more on this topic see www.nursingtimes.net/news/politics/nurses-deliver-scrap-the-cap-pay-petition-to-downing-street/7021762.article.

days because the strikes were between 8am and 5pm) until April of that year. The strike came after protracted negotiations between the British Medical Association (BMA) and NHS Employers, the body that negotiates healthcare employment on behalf of the government, over a new contract for junior doctors. It was the intervention of the then Secretary of State for Health, Jeremy Hunt, in the form of a threat to impose the new contract without the doctors' agreement that precipitated the ballot for strike action in November 2015. The new contracts would abolish most overtime payments and compensate with a rise in the basic pay rate. The BMA claimed that this would result in reduced earnings, particularly for female doctors because the majority of those who worked less than full time were female. Jeremy Hunt claimed that the change was needed to open the way for a seven-day health service, pointing to statistics which he argued indicated an increased death rate for patients admitted to hospital on Saturday or Sunday.[3]

The dispute escalated during the first months of 2016 with junior doctors going as far as withdrawing emergency cover, an unprecedented move in the history of the NHS. Despite this, public support for doctors remained high. A survey undertaken by the Independent newspaper showed that 54% of the public blamed the government for the dispute while only 8% blamed the doctors (Page 2016). In the minds of many, the dispute was about far more than remuneration—it represented a deep distrust felt by many NHS employees and members of the public concerning the Conservative party's real commitment to a free NHS. Many believed that this party, and particularly the Secretary of State, were furthering a covert project of privatising the NHS by a series of financial cuts that would reduce the quality of the service, and the morale of those working within it, to such a degree that the public could be persuaded that drastic action was needed to solve the 'crisis'.

At the time many nurses said, 'today it is the doctors that the government is after; tomorrow it will be us'.

Carol is a nurse in her thirties. I met her at an event where, after hearing her talk, it seemed that she was one of the few nurses who had taken industrial action. I interviewed her a few weeks later. I wanted to find out the circumstances around this unusual act of what I consider courage.

### Tell me about what happened.

So it started with the pay cap and [my nursing friends] began to feel more and more that what we were doing wasn't respected for what it was. We weren't being respected as a profession; we were being seen as sort of handmaidens and, therefore, you could stop paying us as well-educated professionals.

So we felt very… Well, no, actually before I go any further, this is not the people I worked with. This was the problem for me, that a lot of people were just coming into work, doing their job and going home, and the pay cap didn't seem to be affecting them on a

---

3 Many claimed that he misinterpreted statistics that pointed to excess deaths. See the following examples: 'Our nine-point guide to spotting a dodgy statistic' by my favourite statistician David Spiegelhalter at www. theguardian.com/science/2016/jul/17/politicians-dodgy-statistics-tricks-guide. An article in the doctor's magazine *Pulse* suggesting that the difference in weekday and weekend mortality is a statistical artefact: www.pulsetoday. co.uk/news/hot-topics/seven-day-gp-access/excess-deaths-at-weekends-a-statistical-artefact-finds-major-new-study/20031777.article. A detailed but readable blog on statistical sophistication and political intelligence: www.lrb. co.uk/blog/2016/february/jeremy-hunt-s-way-with-statistics.

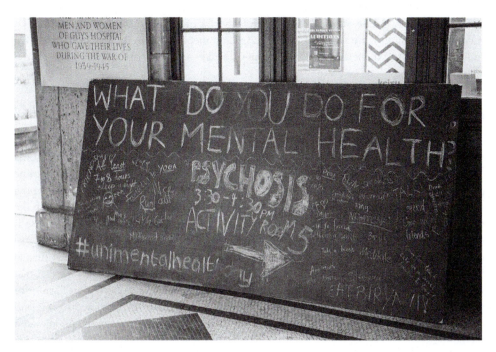

**FIGURE 4.1** A blackboard

day-to-day basis at that time, and it was just going on and on. But in spite of that, enough of us supported and carried out a work-to-rule. It was a bit half-arsed really, to tell the truth. So we came in, we did our job, we didn't do anything extra, we recorded every minute that we worked over our shift—so like 60 minutes if we didn't get a break and every minute that we stayed longer—and we recorded this for a week. Some people really took it seriously, some did it for a couple of days then didn't bother and some people didn't do it at all. And, certainly, where I was working, I know the findings of a survey about unpaid overtime came out and there was a good response rate—it was done by the RCN—and there was a good response rate from our unit. We could see for the first time that we were doing ridiculous numbers of hours over what we were being paid for and, then, still being told that our pay was going to be reduced.

## You were saying that in your trust only some nurses took it up?

Yes, it felt a little bit disappointing. I come from quite a politically active background—my family have always voted, we always talked about politics at home, so I understood what was at stake. My mum used to take me on marches as a girl…

## What particular marches?

So, we would go to the rallies to try and get John Major [Conservative Prime Minister from 1990 to 1997] voted out. So I was very aware of the importance of having a voice, but, actually, we were going in, we were doing the job, we were tired, we didn't really want to be recording every minute of overtime, you know. And there was a lot of apathy in the unit and almost like, 'Oh, you're doing that, are you? Oh, well, I suppose somebody has to do it', and it just all felt really apathetic. And then, we actually went out on strike—not the critical wards—but we did a four-hour strike.

## How did you decide to do that?

There was an RCN ballot, so that was through the union. It was the areas with better team-work, better camaraderie among their colleagues that took this on, like community and some clinics. It was them that you saw on the picket line. I saw a photograph of the picket line just the other day and that was who was on it—believe it or not, there was a rainbow in the background, it had just stopped raining. Because they are working Monday to Friday with the same groups of people, whereas on some acute wards, you work shifts with whoever else is on shift with you, and there was very much a sense on critical care, for example, of, 'well, we can't go out on strike, because we can't leave our patients obviously', and I think that turned into a sense of, 'we don't really care; it's not a real strike, we don't really care'. But the fact that we did, it was massive news—I mean nurses going out on strike; we've been a profession for many, many years and we've never ever been on strike, we've never ever worked to rule and this was the first time ever. And it was all over the news: the nurses, the rain, the puddles and the rainbow.

## So when was this?

This was in 2014. But it all just fell apart; nobody really, in my obstetric unit that is, nobody really felt like anything was going to change—what's the point? Nothing is going to change, we can't go on strike, so what's the point? And then a crucial change happened. About 18 months later the junior doctors stuff kicked off, and the Chair of the BMA was a doctor that had worked with us, so we knew him, and he had left and gone on to somewhere else, and then, the next thing, he pops up as the Chair of the BMA [Chair of the Junior Doctors Committee of the British Medical Association from September 2015 to July 2016]. So we knew him and he had been very… He was always laughing and joking on the ward, we all really liked him, he was a very good doctor and a wonderful obstetrician, really cared about his patients. And so we had this sense of camaraderie with him, hearing him on the media. Actually, I wonder a little if it was a bit that he was a doctor, so we nurses, we fall into that hierarchy a little bit, and it's like, 'Oh, here's a doctor doing it, let's get behind that'. And then the junior doctors' industrial action ramped up and up and got *far* more news coverage than we did, as nurses. And it all began to ramp up and up, and the next thing, they were talking about industrial action, and, actually, everybody across the board was like, 'yep, go for it'. So consultants, all the consultants, covered the junior doctors on the ward, all clinics were cancelled, inductions were cancelled—workload was cancelled, which wasn't done for us. The consultants got behind cancelling workload—and then the nurses got behind covering the workload, so we were doing things, we weren't doing things out of our remit, but we were supporting things that meant you needed less doctors around. So, we did things like increase the elective work the week before and the week after, so that there wouldn't be this kind of, 'oh, you cancelled me'—we didn't want that backlash, so we supported the patients and their families so that they didn't suffer, if you like, so that the doctors were free, to kind of go and do this, and the talk then very much became, 'the junior doctors are doing it for them but they're doing it for all of us, because if they take the doctors, they'll take us next'.

And, actually, although it wasn't our industrial action to take, and it wasn't our message that was being put out there in the media, I understood what they were fighting for. I thought if [the government] can do it for the doctors, they'll have no problem at all washing over the nurses, 'cause they've seen what nurses do when they are offered strike action {laughs}. And so, actually, we put everything we could—I still have my BMA badge on my bag, like, we, as nurses, came to the conclusion that we are all in it together, and if we're not all in it together, we might as well just let them walk all over us. Because, actually, watching the doctors do everything they needed to do and be able to do it, they had a much more powerful voice already—you know, the public hear a nurse and they think, 'what are they up to?' And they hear a doctor and they think 'oh my god, all the doctors are going out, what are we going to do?' So it's like, actually, if we jump behind that, and support that with everything, and they stand as a barrier between the government and the professions that are less well supported by the public—not that they don't love us and all the rest of it. So we did that, and it was just one of the most empowering things I've ever been involved in, I think. It made you see the power that you actually do have, if you all stand up and say, 'actually, that's not alright', and it's not enough for one or two people to say, 'oh, we think this is a good idea', that, actually, if somebody you work with in that way is fighting for something, you have to see the bigger picture and you have to understand that, if they come for them, they'll come for you—don't think, 'oh, well, it's the doctors and they'll be alright, they can look after themselves'.

And the message that was going round the unit all the time was this, that if they can do it [downgrade working conditions] to doctors, they'll definitely do it to us. And people were really rallying around on everything—I mean, our ward was *heaving*, and we had consultants in doing the work of junior doctors. You know, we had one of our consultants—a really quite funny woman in terms of having become a consultant and she would often just sit at the desk and direct her registrars from the desk—just decided she was going to be an SHO [Senior House Officer, a grade of junior doctor now generally known as FY2] for the day, just for fun, and she went round and she couldn't do anything—'I can't do anything: I can't discharge anyone; I don't know the paperwork'. And so she had to learn all of that, all over again, and so, watching her do that was kind of like, 'good for her to show this solidarity'. And we were helping her, even though we probably didn't want to. Yeah, and it just felt like, actually, and when things—ok, they haven't changed but they haven't imposed the things [the contract] that they wanted to in the same way—we felt that was a victory for us, as much as it was for them, because, actually, we're not going to go; we're not just going to let you take the NHS apart and do whatever you like to it, because enough people do still love it and believe in it.

So that was my experience: though my own profession's strike was like, 'oh, well, just' and then, actually, it fuels you to think, 'well, we're a bit rubbish, but actually, we can get behind this much more'. And, I must say, I think it was safe as well, it was a safe way for nurses to get involved in industrial action—because in the media and across the trust it wasn't like, 'Oh, the nurses are on strike'—the overriding message was 'Nurses heroically manage wards while the junior doctors go out on strike'. So we felt, there was a feeling—when I say 'we', I talk about my colleagues and the people around me—that we felt like we had been empowered to support something and it worked, to some extent. So it was interesting.

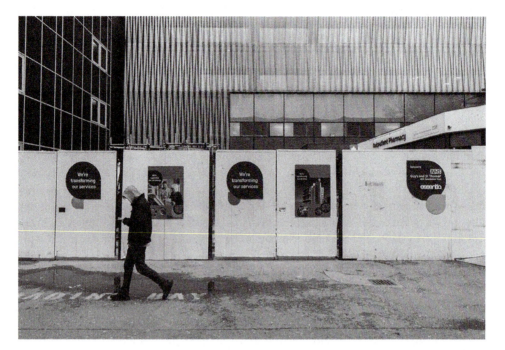

**FIGURE 4.2** Our services

## What was most interesting?

It was about understanding what it was that the junior doctors wanted and what it was that they were fighting for, and a lot of it actually came from them—the discussion was from them about this message of, 'We are one NHS'. Yes, day to day, there is some hierarchy and, day to day, we have issues as two separate professions, but, ultimately, this is about being a cog in the NHS and we are one cog, and if we get taken out, then the rest of you aren't going to work in the same way. And they said things like, 'this is the contract that Jeremy Hunt wants to impose on junior doctors', and it didn't take much to leap from there to realise, 'If they're going to do it you, they're going to do it to us'. And we felt really angry about [media reporting that said] 'junior doctors have these massive salaries and they're spoilt', because, actually, these were people that we worked with day to day and we knew that they didn't, that it was being spun in different ways. And that's really hard, when you see things written about you and your profession, and you just think, that's not true and now the whole world is reading this, that's awful. And so, there was definitely that thing— we felt an obligation to be part of this. The members of the BMA that were trying to get people involved were saying, 'this is bigger than just us, there is something bigger going on here', and they felt very strongly it wasn't just them. They believed that this was part of an underhand way of starting to dismantle the NHS and weaken the professions, and I don't know if it's true or borne out, but that's what it felt like. Definitely. And I do feel that the NHS is under attack, so you have to defend it. Nurses can be very good at complaining and doing nothing.

### So what were the managers like at that time? Managers are in a difficult position—or can be.

The nurse managers, I think, just started managing us; you know, they just started dealing with the workload and I don't remember any of them being vocal about anything or saying anything, but they certainly didn't cast opinion on people for choosing to get involved in the action or otherwise. I definitely feel that we were supported to support them, so we did just get on with managing the workload, and people worked hard—the consultants and nurse managers worked together to make sure that work was distributed properly. Actually, I remember one of our patients said she was laughing because she'd said, 'I was really worried when I heard the doctors were going on strike because, oh my goodness, what if something happens during my operation?' And she was laughing because she ended up with a nurse manager as her nurse and two consultants, in fact, three consultants if you include the anaesthetist, as her care team, alongside the other nursing staff and she said, 'this strike's great!' She was thrilled that she got better, not better care, but obviously more senior care, 'cause the managers were on the floor helping us out. Yeah, I remember she had gone from panic to incredulous disbelief—like, 'got consultant this and consultant that and manager this'. So our managers were very supportive.

### It's good to hear stories like that, because sometimes it seems they are few and far between.

And I still think there's a long way to go, isn't there? We're never going to know what the government really wants and what they're doing—you can only just take these battles one at a time and hope for the best, I think. My eyes were certainly opened by this. It was a complicated story but the conditions were right for us to change. This was an interesting time in my life. I will never be the same, that's for sure.

# 5

# BEVERLEY, THE STUDENT NURSE WHO REFUSED TO FEAR

Beverley is a student nurse who told me about her 'ah-ha' moment. It was to do with fear, or rather, her refusal of fear. And what she told me brought about a sudden realisation of my own.

Beverley is in her early thirties and so would be considered a mature student, even in nursing where the numbers of students aged 25 and over had been rising until the withdrawal of the NHS bursary in England from 2017.[1] Like some other mature students, Beverley looks after small children so, needless to say, getting to lectures and clinical placements on time can involve complicated and sometimes precarious arrangements. But then the NHS, as well as universities, have family-friendly policies and adapt their approaches to ensure that students like Beverley—and qualified nurses—are not disadvantaged. Before starting her training as a nurse, Beverley had a career, she told me, working from home and importing unusual fashion accessories including jewellery made from sliced Barbie doll parts.[2] Working from home can be conducive to childcare although it can lead to its own pressures that require imaginative solutions. But she gave this up because she wanted to nurse. The decision, however, was not without cost:

> I just feel constantly exhausted and guilty. Getting to the uni can take two hours each way, on a bad day. I constantly feel like I'm letting my kids down. It breaks my heart sometimes when I have to leave before the little one wakes up and come back when he's already in bed, sometimes two days in a row. I don't think placements are family friendly at all. Although I know I will never get this time back with them, finishing the course means we can have a stable and secure future.

---

1  See the Health Foundation's report *Rising Pressure: the NHS Workforce Challenge* by Buchan, Charlesworth et al. (2017). Some details are available at www.health.org.uk/chart-change-profile-nursing-students-england. Placed applicant numbers of 20–24 year olds dropped by 9% in 2017, while numbers of applicants aged 25 years and more dropped by 11% after rising steadily since 2013. Commentators believe that this reflects older would-be applicants' reluctance to take on the personal debt involved in student loans.

2  If you think this is implausible, check this article on a similar product: www.telegraph.co.uk/news/newstopics/howaboutthat/3488857/Sliced-Barbie-dolls-become-sinister-fashion-accessory.html. Barbie was launched as long ago as 1959 by American toy company Mattel. If you have a Barbie and want to help her into a career as a Registered Nurse, see https://barbie.mattel.com/shop/en-us/ba/bill-greening/registered-nurse-barbie-doll-r4472.

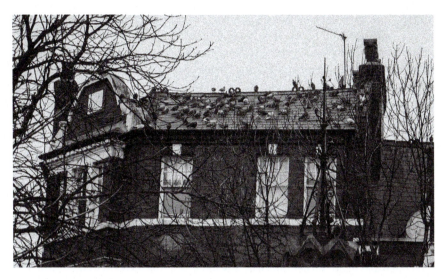

**FIGURE 5.1** The birds

A BSc nursing course in the UK currently takes three years to complete. Among those who teach these courses, there is an accepted wisdom that the second year is a difficult one for students. Because of this, many courses include a module at the start of Year Two specially designed to help students look back constructively on what they had learned in the first year and to evaluate their expectations of the year that lies ominously ahead. There are almost endless opportunities to support students in creative ways, though most of these are lost. It was during the first session of a module like this that Beverley's story starts. She wrote a detailed account, full of quotations from her lecturer, in an email to me and I later travelled up to the Midlands city where she studied to discuss her unsettling but ultimately liberating experience. The story that follows of her discovery of a particular kind of resilience is taken both from our conversation and her written words.

## Beverley's story

Most of our set love our tutor and see her as a kind of Mother figure. She calls us 'ladies', even though there is a man in the class. I must ask him what he thinks about that. She is good at setting ground rules, at her best, I'd say. Every class needs rules:

'If your lips are moving, I can tell. If your lips are moving, I will have to stop the class. Now, ladies, you are starting Year Two. How do you feel about that?'

One person says 'excited'. Maureen [the tutor] says, 'That's good', and, sounding a bit like a medium at a séance asks, 'What other feelings am I getting?'

Others call out from the three rows of desks, 'I'm scared', 'I'm anxious'. Maureen repeats the words carefully and asks the class, 'Why?' Everyone, mostly everyone, is usually quick to answer her questions. But this time no one offers an answer. Instead, a noisy bus goes by on the wet road in heavy rain outside. Someone else calls out, 'I want to cry'. Maureen summarises while she walks at the front of the classroom. 'OK. It's about being unsure and it's about coping. Having been a student myself, of course I know where you are coming from, but things have changed a lot, believe me. You are going to feel…certain things.'

Some love the way we know that she can empathise with us and we know, from the hints she has made, that she has been through tough times.

'As a nurse myself, I have had to study throughout my career. There is mandatory training—do you know what that means? You have to complete that—and competency-based training. The NMC will make sure.'

Whenever Maureen talks about 'The NMC' it always feels like a warning, even though some of us are not quite sure what the NMC is or what the letters stand for. Someone joked that it stands for Nurses Must Care. But the class always goes very quiet when Maureen mentions the NMC. Maureen never has a problem getting our attention.

'Get into groups of four or five—not six. I want you to nominate one person to write on my flip chart. The question I want you to answer is "What advice would you give a student starting Year One?" I want you to think back to what you would have wanted someone with more experience to say to you'.

We discuss it in our rows of desks. Getting up would have been easier, but Maureen slips between the lines to hover over each group in turn. When she is ready, she pulls the top off her marker pen and stands by her flip chart. I wonder why she asked us to nominate someone to write. Perhaps she forgot or just thought it easier to do it herself. Someone suggests, 'Be assertive'. Maureen's marker is poised above the paper but she turns around and looks at us. Another bus goes by.

'Is assertive the word you want to use, or another word?' My fellow student is silent, a little confused. Maureen explains, 'I want you to be absolutely clear that it is unsafe practice to work on your own. You need to be absolutely clear about that. This is protected time for your learning.' Maureen turns away and writes 'COMMUNICATION' on the flip chart, then turns round to give us more advice.

'If you appear disinterested or switched off on placement, what will happen? Will mentors want to teach you? What do you think?'

All: 'No.'

'Is there anything else anyone wants to tell me?'

There is silence. She often makes points by asking questions.

'I was hoping for something else, that you would tell me something different, but maybe that will come up later in discussion.'

I sense we are searching hard in our heads for that 'something else' that Maureen wants. Each of us wants to be the one that says it. How could we be so slow to understand what she wants from us? But Maureen has already moved on.

'Setting boundaries and rules is something you would do well to remember throughout your career. Don't self-sacrifice. You will burn out. Do you know about burnout?'

No one does and Maureen explains its different components. Depersonalisation is one. The others I don't remember.

One student then tells an anecdote of a near miss in a placement—I don't remember the details. Maureen listens and draws a lesson from it. She tells her about the NMC guidelines and gives a warning about practising beyond our level of knowledge. She tells us, 'No nurse administers a drug without that little bit of fear. You have to question everything you do', i.e. concentrate hard and check everything endlessly. I can feel the class becoming silent and tense, but the next topic starts and there is relieved laughter.

Maureen explains the grading system for our work in Year Two and how failed work is dealt with. She gives us some simple advice: 'Pass the first time'. She gives us lots of advice about how to organise our time for working using her own experience as an example. We ask for lots of information about the course, particularly about what happens to students who fail.

A couple of the students are talking. Maureen stops the class: 'You can't care for patients safely if you don't use the information that I am giving you now. They will test you, they will put you through your paces if you don't know your stuff.' The class is silent again, wondering who exactly is the 'they'. Is it the NMC? Is it other nurses?

'OK, in Year Two, what do you think you need to take responsibility for?' Maureen asks the class. There are some answers up already on a slide.

'Learning.' 'OK—there are people talking in the class. It's disrespectful. If you want to talk leave the room…' She tells a cautionary tale about professional standards and a particular student she has come across.

'What else do you need to take responsibility for?'

'Time management'. 'So why don't we do it?'

Instead of a reply, someone asks a question about the right way of taking blood pressure. Maureen doesn't explore what's at work in this random question and provides the answer. But it seems to satisfy the student. There is a pause.

'You are very quiet for a change!', says Maureen.

'It's because there is so much to think about', some of us say.

'It's not over yet—I still have more to tell you.' Maureen explains about failure. Someone asks a nervous question. Maureen says, 'Listen—you need to listen carefully.' We tell her that it is daunting. Maureen has the information that we need in order to know how to pass. 'Make sure you don't miss those first few days of Year Two'—you will be shooting yourself in the foot if you do.'

But then she moves onto a topic that makes my heart suddenly race. 'In Year Two, it's a 9am start. That means your bottoms need to be on the seats then. If you are *one minute* late, we will not let you in. There is no 'ten minute' rule.' She pronounces 'ten minute' as if it were some foolish indulgence given to spoilt children.

I have to speak out, more from anxiety than courage: 'Sorry, but that is not always possible, Maureen.'

'Well, that means missing input…' is her answer.

'But could you not consider work–life balance—?'

'Let's face reality', interrupts Maureen. She sticks with the rule. 'I'm not unsympathetic with those who have got families but my job is to teach you in these modules. OK? It's as simple as that. Right, let's move on, shall we? So what advice would you give a student starting Year Two?'

Much of the input from the other students from then onwards sounds like they are saying the right thing, 'be punctual', etc. I realise that Maureen has the authority to tell us how things are. Most of my classmates seem to have already accepted this. I can't remember when or how that happened.

'You need a break now.' There is a sigh of relief from the class.

During the break I make my way outside, while most of the rest of the class go the other way to get coffee. I need to make a call to check on my children. My hands are shaking a little bit. I noticed, while listening for the call to connect, that the rain was stopping. The disappointment I felt that I was not being listened to grew quickly. It reminded me of a bruise under the skin. My respect and admiration for Maureen drained away in those few moments. Suddenly, I understood why students leave. I understood why the dreaded Year Two was so feared and difficult. In Year One, despite the shocks, you are still propelled by your desire of wanting to be a nurse. In Year Three, the end is not far off. Now I was asking myself, 'what have I got myself into?' I was probably standing outside for less than five minutes, but in that time everything changed. Even my body felt different.

Beverley continued, telling me about her later thoughts and discoveries.

Once I dared to say that I found this approach oppressive, bit by bit I began to learn that other members of my class also found Maureen frightening, and not just Maureen. I was not alone. Realising this became the first move in putting myself together, back together but different this time. It occurred to me that so much of the tone of our teaching is of warnings, maintaining that slight level of fear. Perhaps some tutors have learned that sustaining a certain amount of anxiety is a useful way of keeping student attention and engagement in the course, as well as class discipline. I am sure that if you challenged those same tutors about this they would be shocked. I can't believe that any tutor in a caring occupation would come to their work with such a personality issue that they would want to make students frightened. Or be so uninterested in the impact they are having on us. But there is a real power imbalance. The teacher has the information that we need to know about how to pass. And everyone wants to pass. Maybe, if a tutor keeps a certain amount of fear in the room, they can dip into the role of saviour when they wish to and get an emotional reward from that. Maybe some of them miss having patients that they could make feel better. They sometimes tell us that we need to be resilient, but if they changed their approach to teaching we wouldn't need to be quite so resilient in the first place.

## Reflections on critical pedagogy

By the time we met, Beverley had gathered material for an article she and some colleagues had started to write about student experiences and teaching styles—such was the power of her experience in that classroom and the realisation that it had brought. What had started as an assignment about critical thinking ended up with a discovery, partly by chance, of descriptions of 'critical pedagogy' and that was the starting point for their article and thinking.

While critical thinking courses set out to teach students how to spot faulty logic and other inadequate truth claims, like research findings that do not flow from the data collected, critical pedagogy is more fundamentally critical. And critical pedagogy provided Beverley with a theoretical account of her experience and that of her classmates. It is, in that sense, more holistic than learning critical thinking skills and offers more potential to act as a basis for action and change. So, what do we mean by 'critical pedagogy'? We can start with the questions posed by the critical theorists of the Frankfurt School, and others, about how society—capitalist society—manages to maintain itself as the only imaginable way of organising society.[3] The concept of ideology grew up as a term to describe one way that powerful classes can reinforce their position of dominance over those who are dominated. For Karl Marx, those who own and control the means of production can use their accumulated wealth to enhance, maintain and expand their power. One of the ways they can do this is through ideological power or control over how people think about the nature of the social world and their own place in it. Marx developed the notion of what we call hegemony, 'leadership with the consent of

3 For a highly readable summary of critical theory, the Frankfurt School and the ideas of Karl Marx, see Chapter 8 in my previous book *Critical Resilience for Nurses* (Traynor 2017).

the led', to describe this. The ruling class can establish and maintain its hegemony over other classes through the use of force, for example through the police, but also by means of ideology and socialisation via the media and, in our case, the education system. A follower of Marx, Louis Althusser called these forms of control 'Ideological State Apparatuses' (Althusser 1971). One strong feature of ideology is that it offers a compelling and broad picture of how things are and couples this with offering the individual a place within that world. Traditionally, the operation of ideology has been said to keep oppressed workers, the class that Marx called the proletariat, from turning against their oppressors, the owners of the means of production. Education systems play a prominent part in this by offering some kind of financial rewards bound up with systems of conformity enacted in testing, tracking and subtle and not so subtle approaches to socialisation. Critical pedagogy first sets out to recognise the way that traditional education can perpetuate and reinforce inequality in the name of education or of providing opportunity. Think of the 'Windrush' generation of black workers encouraged into second-class Enrolled Nurse training that satisfied the need for workers to staff the early UK NHS while keeping them at a level of work with no opportunity for career advancement.[4] Critical pedagogy not only refuses to engage in such mechanisms to maintain an economic, social and racist status quo but also sets out to open students' eyes to their own disadvantage and to encourage and enable them to act to change it. We could use the word 'empower', though that term, in typical ideological fashion, has been used to describe and promote its own opposite, a state where students (or others) are structurally disempowered and then urged to take personal responsibility for their situation. Berbules and Berk describe critical pedagogy in this way:

> It is an effort to work within educational institutions and other media to raise questions about inequalities of power, about the false myths of opportunity and merit for many students, and about the way belief systems become internalized to the point where individuals and groups abandon the very aspiration to question or change their lot in life.
>
> *Burbules and Berk 1999*

The founders and advocates of critical pedagogy were often directly involved with political struggle—against the interests of large corporations and the governments that supported them. Paulo Freire, for example, worked originally promoting adult literacy among Latin American peasant communities (see Freire 1970) before his work was taken up more internationally. Critical pedagogy in nurse education has different, though similar, emphases. Those who promote it acknowledge the operation of power on and within the profession. For example, Sue Dyson writes:

> Conventional pedagogy such as [nurse education] is characterised by the need to transmit… skills, facts and standards of moral and social conduct considered necessary and is imposed from above and outside… Nurse teachers are the instrument by which nursing knowledge is conveyed and behaviours consistent with nursing are enforced.
>
> *Dyson 2018, p. 69*

---

4 Enrolled nurses were known as 'second-level' nurses. The training was introduced in the 1940s and phased out in the mid-1980s. 'Demand for a statutorily recognised second-level nursing qualification began in the 1930s, when hospitals were unable, or unwilling, to recruit 'expensive' registered nurses, and were making increased use of various types of unqualified aides and assistants' (Seccombe, Smith et al. 1997).

Dyson believes that the revelation and publicity around the now well-known poor care at Stafford hospital forced both the English Department of Health and the regulator (the NMC) to take measures to control recruitment to and the content of nurse education more closely. Key to this was a drive toward a kind of standardisation.

But a critical pedagogic approach will also involve asking, 'Do the structures of our education work for the benefit of certain groups while tending to put barriers in the way of others?' By structures, I mean particular entrance or attendance requirements, or examples used in teaching, or styles of teaching, or the social class and ethnic characteristics of those who teach. It is hard to know where 'structure' ends and 'agency' starts[5] but within the practice of educators we may notice a tendency toward 'microaggression', the casual degradation of a marginalised group by (perhaps well-meaning, perhaps not) members of a more 'mainstream' group (Sue 2010). Does the way that 'professional' and 'unprofessional' appearance or behaviour is encouraged or censured reflect a cultural bias on the part of those with the power to impose such rules?

Just as the critical theorists asked how maintaining ideological dominance worked to support the smooth working of capitalist society, we can ask, 'How do the implicit ideologies repeated within nurse education support, perhaps in complex and perverse ways, the smooth running of health services?' Historically, maintaining a tradition of fear that perpetuated a certain subservience within nursing was perhaps essential to the profession's early hegemonic and heavily gendered relationship with medicine (Freidson 1970). Perhaps it also ensured that new recruits were likely to be pliable to the instructions of nurses above them in professional hierarchies. So the apparent maintenance of fear and tantalising refusal to encourage confidence and independent thinking that Beverley described can be understood as having this function. That is, perhaps, a structural explanation. But Beverley also asked whether an individual educator would consciously adopt this approach and concluded that it was unlikely. More likely, she thought, is that many nurse lecturers have a strong sense of professional tradition and, therefore, often bring their own experiences as nurses into the classroom, sometimes as pedagogical material and sometimes for other reasons. And if those experiences were of their own fear and lack of confidence, then it would be natural to draw on these negative patterns when dealing with a class of students. It could, as Beverley perceptively noted, provide certain emotional rewards, similar to those that a nurse still at the bedside might reap from providing reassurance to frightened patients.

Beverley's story both shocked me and felt strangely familiar. As she pointed out, the particular pedagogical style that she encountered was not the norm where she studied, by any means, but it was not a singular event. Beverley, alongside some of her fellow students, found that this event provided the foundation to a raising of consciousness among some of the class. They worked together on an article that relates their experiences to theories of critical pedagogy. They also put in a complaint to the institution where they were studying. At the time of writing, the outcome of their complaint is not known.

---

5 Agency and structure are two fundamental sociological concepts. *Structure* is said to be the long-standing patterned arrangements that influence or limit choices and opportunities available. *Agency* is the capacity of individuals to act independently and to make their own free choices (https://en.wikipedia.org/wiki/Structure_and_agency).

# 6

# LAURA, STUDENT NURSES AND 'REAL' NURSES

> When you go out there and see the real nurses, the registered ones… they're physically there but their minds and hearts are not really for caring.

In medieval times, novices who joined monasteries, nunneries and religious orders went through initiation rites. Their heads were shaved, they started wearing strange and uncomfortable clothes and the names that they had lived with from birth, the names that their mothers had given them, were exchanged for new ones. These practices enacted the loss of a previous life and the beginning of a fundamentally new identity. In some ways, daunting coursework and the extremes of anxiety experienced in early clinical settings, sometimes with little apparent support from staff, perform the same kind of function for nurses. The unfamiliarity and terror make you highly susceptible to professional socialisation, that is, to put it simply, wanting to gain approval and fit in. This kind of workplace regime, whether achieved as a deliberate strategy or more as a result of lack of time, can also bring about extremely close bonds between novices. Often those bonds can give rise to peer-group norms that are based on a strong critique of those in authority.

This chapter tells the story of Laura. It is about a student nurse's difficult relationship with the qualified nurses that she worked with and relied on for her own registration. It is based partly on a discussion during a focus group that I ran in 2015 with third year nursing students and partly on a conversation with Laura about two years after the original group. Laura looks back on her time as a student and comments on the original group discussion. Like many other stories in this collection, the focus is on the personal transformation that can occur following rigorous analysis of the causes of what resilience researchers describe as 'adversity'.

'I had always been interested in anatomy and physiology and had worked as a beauty therapist and then specialised in complementary therapy. I was doing a herbal medicine degree and, at the end of it, I decided that I wanted to do something practical and also helpful. I tried some voluntary work on a medical ward in my local hospital, which was an eye-opener. After the first time, I went home shaken by what I had seen and smelt, that mixture of disinfectant and incontinence. After the second time, I was on a complete high because I discovered "I can cope with this." I applied to train and was accepted. In the meantime, I worked as a healthcare assistant [HCA] in a rehab unit for people after stroke or major head injury. It was a very low-pressure job, though I remember the ward sister there was a real old-school nurse and was cruel to some of the older female patients. But overall it was relaxed and there was scope to be mischievous. I remember another HCA and I, along with a patient, a young man who had a major head injury after trying to kill himself by jumping in front of a truck, locked ourselves in a tiny store cupboard, and the other HCA and I went through the alphabet with words that described our situation: awful, bizarre, claustrophobic, derisory, excessive… The guy loved it. He couldn't speak but he was killing himself laughing. When I started training, things changed abruptly. Some of the lecturers could be a bit old school, but the staff nurses often seemed to be taking out their frustrations on students, the only people they actually had any power over, the only people they weren't frightened of.'

Other nurses in Laura's group had been keen to talk about witnessing approaches to care that, they said, shocked them:

> Delyse: I mean, since starting the journey, right back from the access course, before I'd had any placement experience, before starting the degree, because you kind of tend to notice the environment more when you are in a medical setting—like one of my parents was in hospital—you tend to notice bad practice…
>
> Ini: …or bad communication or no empathy, so it was right when we were in there doing our access course that it was, that started to niggle at me, like, well, 'I don't want to be like that, I want to change the system', albeit whether that's going to happen is another story for after, but it's seeing bad and poor practice that inspired me to definitely push to get onto the course.
>
> Michael: Does anybody else have that feeling?
>
> Many voices: Yeah.
>
> Ini: Yeah, I was definitely, it's seeing, you know, old-school nurses who can't be bothered. They're biding their time until their pension comes up {general laughter}. Yeah, that's what it is, that's what it is! They think they know better than the rest, you know, and it's looking at those, it's, 'I don't want to be like that and I don't want the system, I don't want the NHS to be full of staff just like that.'
>
> Sabryna: It's like the caring aspect that's missing, being empathetic and being nice to the patient, and just talking to the patient, that sort of side of care, that's what's lacking. I've seen nurses who don't have that side of the care but just have the technical side, so, for example, they're doing the caring but they're not showing the patient any, I don't know, what's the word, empathy.
>
> Ini: It's just the attitude that these nurses carry, 'cause it's like, we go in there, we're so shocked by some of the things that we've seen, and I say to myself I would never do that, and they turn to you and say, 'just wait till you qualify. You say you're not going to do this and you're not going to do that but you will', and it's quite sad that that's the attitude that they carry. So what are you trying to say—we shouldn't be caring for these patients; we should just be doing it because it's a job?
>
> Michael: Can you tell me a bit more about that?
>
> Ini: So it's like some of these nurses, they just do it because it's a job; they know they're going to get paid at the end of it, so they're not necessarily doing it because they have that caring attitude and they really want to do it 'cause they want to help someone. We go in there as students and we're observing what they're doing and how they're caring for these patients. Where's the caring aspect that you're supposed to be showing to this patient?

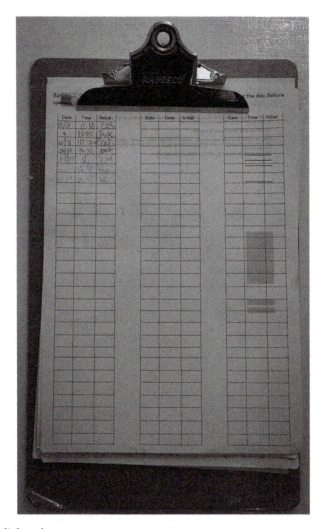

**FIGURE 6.1** A clipboard

Laura was not so confident that she understood the motivation of the staff nurses she encountered during training or about students necessarily maintaining a principled position once qualified:

'To me it seemed that so many nurses—there are exceptions who are fantastic—don't have any awareness of the effect they are having on people, whether they are the patients, other nurses or students. And they—some—don't seem remotely interested in reflecting on that. They do seem to be prodded by fear though, fear of doctors who can treat them witheringly or of more senior nurses, who themselves seem frightened of someone above them. And that lack of self-awareness… This would be funny if it weren't so sad—someone, a student, who was one cohort ahead of us throughout, she was very critical of staff nurses, with a lot of the stuff you have heard in our group. I bumped into her in the canteen the next day after she had qualified and become a staff nurse. She was holding court about how terrible students are and how they know nothing, are poorly motivated and how they waste your time with their questions. That was the very next day. I remember in our focus group some of the class saying how the nurses would say to them "You just wait till you are qualified—you will change your approach." They had some bravado saying that they would uphold empathy once they were qualified, but the fact that they talked about it so much shows you how worried they were.'

Ini: I think losing your empathy is learned behaviour because I can guarantee that somebody who's been qualified two years is still going to be as empathetic as us watching. Someone who's been in the job fifteen or twenty years isn't. It's learned behaviour and, unfortunately, it's the stresses of the budget, staff reductions…

Kimona: But why should we allow that to interfere?

Ini: We shouldn't, it's not right. It's not right, which is why, when we're fifteen years down the line, we shouldn't let it affect us. So when we qualify and go on the ward, and we're the goody two shoes going around, making sure we're empathetic and caring, every single one of us is going to be the one with the fifteen-years nurse on our backs, saying, 'you haven't done your care plans', 'you're not on time with your meds', 'they can get to the toilet themselves', 'they can wait for that cup of tea'. And it's learned behaviour—you can't help but think, 'do you know what, they're not going to die if they don't have that cup of tea; I do need to do my care plan.' But being empathetic…

Kimona: But I think once you're working there, everybody tends to carry that attitude…

Sabryna: Being empathetic is making that cup of tea for that person. They don't care about their care plan.

Ini: I think we, going in as new nurses, as newly qualified nurses, we need to know that, let's carry this attitude where we won't be like them in fifteen years' time.

Sabryna: But saying that…

Kimona: We're going to try—I know it's hard…

Laura continued:

'The experience [of being a student nurse] drained me of my identity. It was a powerful mix of feeling horrified by what you see. I remember early in my training, neurosurgery, people with huge bandages on their heads who couldn't speak. Being paralysed with fear because of lack of knowledge—I didn't know what to do. I didn't know why the patients were there or what had happened to them. So that kind of horror and complete disorientation made me totally vulnerable, so if the nurses ignored me or were sharp or impatient with me or made a joke at my expense, I couldn't stand up for myself or question them. That was the second part of the mix. And I would be in that state for shift after shift. Sometimes to even get any words out of my mouth at all was an achievement. Added to that, of course, you knew you had to be signed off on the placements, but I almost never even thought about that, I was so focused on just surviving each shift.'

'What do you mean by being drained of identity?'

'I got married half way into the course, in Year Two, I think. My husband had nothing to do with nursing or healthcare. One evening, I remember, he put his arms around me and told me that he loved me and I just winced inside because I felt completely worthless and unworthy of anybody loving me. I couldn't tell him that. In fact, I felt that my own worthlessness infected him too and that he was tainted for loving me. It was as if all the nurses I had had to work with were in the room smirking at him from the shadows. It was a really dark and horrible feeling. Terrible that working in that environment and with those people had brought me to a place like that.'

'You say that you think the whole environment was full of fear. It's clear that you were certainly frightened.'

'Yes, perhaps I saw fear everywhere because I was looking through the eyes of fear. The eyes of Laura Mars! I have often thought that my colleagues who saw lack of caring and empathy for patients everywhere were wanting some caring for themselves—from the nurses.'

In the focus group, someone did mention a lack of resources and staff reductions as one cause of poor care. Nobody followed it up. In fact, someone said that it should not affect the way that nurses care for patients.

'Yes, it is about resources and overwork, of course, but I think there were also more hidden things going on that had a big effect on how we were treated. That was to do with lack of power and fear. Perhaps my own fear gave me a special insight into the fear of the nurse. I started following it up with some reading. I read about horizontal violence to start with.'

'Which is?'

'Well, if you type the term into a search engine, all of the results on the first page are about nursing, which shows you who is talking about it, but it didn't start there. What some nurses forget is that the key to horizontal violence is that it is displaced violence directed against one's peers, rather than adversaries. It started with post-colonial writers like Albert Memmi, who wrote about the psychological effects of being among a colonised group. His book on this subject was published in the 1950s.[1] He, or perhaps another writer,[2] talks about how the oppressed can identify with the oppressor and despise their own culture. And someone else talks about how the oppressed can actually become afraid of freedom. Maybe for some nurses there is some level of fear of taking responsibility.'

Some of the group had talked about bullying:

Sabryna: There's a lot of… You will see things and a lot of [nurses] will just keep quiet because they're scared about raising their concerns, you know, otherwise, they get picked on—you can easily get bullied in working and I've seen it.

Ini: Yeah, I've seen people…

Sabryna: Either you just do as they, do as the Jones' do, or just don't come to work; it's as simple as that.

Michael: How does that work? You say there's bullying.

Sabryna: Well, I don't know whether I should go down the line as saying bullying, but there's people, as you rightly explain, they see it just as a job, but a lot of them, you know what I mean, sometimes, they might want to raise concerns but we [unintelligible] at the end of the day. You whistle blow on them, what happens to your career, next thing you know, you get pushed out of a job.

Ini: Driven out…

Sabryna: You have to be careful how you go about with stuff like that. People don't like to hear the truth when it comes to the healthcare, it's like you just get picked on, you're the worst person ever and that type of thing, but it's there. You see it at work, you see it at placement, you know, whenever you go to work, it is there. I've seen it myself, just like you guys so…

1 Like Albert Camus, Memmi wrote fiction, but the book Laura is referring to is *The Colonizer and the Colonized* (Memmi [1957] 1991).
2 I think Laura is thinking of Paulo Freire, who is mentioned in Chapter 5 about the student who refused fear. Fear seems to be a theme here.

Michael: So it's seems to be a general kind of—nobody's disagreeing with this.

All: No. {Laughter}

The group also talked about what could be considered to be aspects of horizontal violence. I had asked them what they looked forward to once qualified:

Kimona: I think implementing changes…

Laura: That will be a very good thing, and obviously when you're qualified, I will talk a bit more…

Sabryna: …outspoken.

Ini: I will definitely be like, 'this is not on'. Like you, 'this is not on—obviously there are policies here, you're not following them, so I don't want to talk about it again' sort of thing. I would implement change definitely. As students, it's very hard.

Joanna: Just to be treated equally.

Laura: You're treated like you're nothing really…

{Lots of speaking simultaneously.}

Joanna: They don't treat you like a person. They don't even call you by your name. Look—I have a name!

{Many interruptions.}

Sabryna: I don't think newly qualified nurses are treated as equals though. I've just seen newly qualified nurses just being put down a lot; even more than us student nurses…

Ini: Yeah, but you know what—it's down to the individual to speak out. 'Cause, you know what, as far as I'm concerned, you could be working for five years but me and you are the same. I don't have the same knowledge as you but treat me as an equal. And that's what you need to express to these people when you go out there as a qualified nurse. And then they can't treat you as though you are insignificant.

Laura continued on the theme of internalised oppression:

'I read a blog written by a prisoner in America on this topic.[3] He said something like, "one sign that an oppressed person has a 'fear of freedom' can be their personal preference for gregarious friendship, rather than for real comradeship. The only conception that this oppressed person has of freedom is a desire for the oppressor's 'freedom' to oppress." I'm not sure how you can tell the difference between those two types of relationship—'true' or just gregarious—but the second part is true to my experience of being a student nurse.'

In the group, Laura and her fellow students voiced strong views about how certain relationships 'on the ward' could leave them feeling an excluded outsider:

Ini: What could you really do, you as an individual that's coming onto a new ward and you've got this group of people and they've already formed relationships, they've formed their friendships. If anything happens, you know that one's gonna stick up for that one; they're not gonna have your back 'cause they don't know you and it takes a long time to settle in with that team.

---

3 Laura appears to be referring to 4STRUGGLEMAG and this article in particular: https://4strugglemag.org/2010/07/23/examining-the-internalized-oppressor-complex/.

Laura: But I think if I entered a place like that I would probably be trying to get good relationships with the team that I work with and then, from then, I would just be challenging or moving, or changing things slowly, slowly because you can't just be, go to the ward and say, 'ok, I don't agree with this' and people would start like…

Ini: How will you cope though? You go to a ward, see something you're not happy with, even if it's just a comment to a patient or another member of staff, and you report it or you pull them up on it and then you're deemed the outsider, you're deemed the stirrer and you're then the outsider of the group, every shift, you're excluded. How do you deal with that as a human being, not just as a nurse, as a human being; thinking back to when you were in school, if you weren't in the in-crowd and, you know, even out with your friends, if you're not always the lively one, how do you deal with that?

Laura: Well, I guess it's quite hard, it's quite hard to deal with that…

Ini: It's impossible!

Laura: But, um…

Sabryna: You have to be thick skinned.

Ini: Yeah, you need, I think you need to have a good approach…

Sabryna: And if we were in the army, fair enough; we're not, we're supposed to be in a caring profession and we're doing that to each other.

I showed Laura the transcript of this part of the discussion. It brought back memories for her.

'Hum! What's interesting is how they did the very thing they were condemning, my old colleagues—they excluded my view about how it might be possible to constructively change practice and influence culture. I just gave up trying to get my view across. And it doesn't give me much hope that they are going to be that different to the nurses they are complaining about here. It's also an example of being gregarious rather than comradely!'

'So what happened after that focus group? It was near the end of Year Three, wasn't it?'

'We finished the course and nearly everyone passed—I passed. I went to work in another place. It was OK. I was pleased to have passed. I'd started so many other things and not followed them through. I was determined to make something of this. I worked my first job in another rehab unit. Like my first experience as an HCA, I found this a relaxed place. But then I trained to be a health visitor because I wanted to get out into a slightly more expansive environment. I drive a little car around north London. There's some scope for community-based work, which I like, and I do some health promotion with a school nurse in our local primary school.'

'What do you think today about the issues that you discussed in the focus group?'

'I think students do have better experiences than we did—even just a few years later. When I talk to the student nurses who come out with me today, it seems that they find that most qualified nurses are genuinely trying to help and support them but are just so overwhelmed by work that they find it difficult. I think it is important to try to see the bigger picture and, if it does seem that 'the real nurses' are treating you badly, the chances are that it's not personal and that they are caught up in their own response to an underfunded health service or professional frustrations. That would definitely be my advice to a student today—don't take it personally. Understand the big picture.'

# 7

## POLLY, THE NURSE WHO WROTE POETRY AND WENT MISSING

Polly was a nurse who was a poet. It is not unusual to come upon poetry written by nurses.[1] Perhaps some need the space from involvement in the highly charged world of sickness that counting syllables and searching for rhymes can provide. Things went better for Polly as a poet than as a nurse.

The trick with poetry, she told me during our interview in 2016, is creating the illusion of being spoken to by the author, naturally and spontaneously. But writing is full of lies. It was clear that she knew a great deal more in 2016 than she did years earlier when she had started nurse training, both about nursing and about writing poetry. After she had done academically well in a girls' school in west London, an illness that remained a slight mystery during our interview emerged, purely coincidentally she said, at the time of her A-level exams. It seemed that her brief experience at the receiving end of healthcare at this crucial time opened up a curiosity for her about what it would feel like to be responsible for its delivery. 'Almost too easily', she said, she imagined the possibility of 'making a difference'. After briefly researching options in healthcare training, she applied for a nursing course at an institution close to where she was living with her parents at that time. She was accepted to start later the same year. It was clear from our interview that, like many new nurses in training, she was idealistic, drawn by the imagined one-to-one relationship with a patient.

'I think I wanted to do nursing—I wanted to do something rewarding—and I'm good with people, I like to mix with people, um, you know, I'm quite caring by nature so it just fitted who I am really.'

Again, like many other students, she had to adapt her preconceptions about nurses to the reality of her daily experience.

'So the idea of nurses wasn't exactly what I thought. But, at the beginning, I did think it was something quite negative, 'cause I thought nurses should always be nice, so why are some of them like this, and, as you go along, you actually understand, you need to actually be assertive. Obviously, don't be rude, but being too nice and being passive actually doesn't help, so I've learned that, 'cause me, I was quite a passive, nice-ish person, I think; I was quite timid…'

---

1  See http://www.rattle.com/when-the-poet-happens-to-be-a-nurse-by-madeleine-mysko/.

But I was struck that trauma seemed to follow close on the heels of this idealism, this sensitivity, or rather was its flip side. Polly talked to me about an early experience during a first year placement:

'I remember I was shaken to the core after being sent to theatre for the first time. There was an operation for bladder cancer—advanced cancer, the first operation I'd ever seen. I won't tell you what they did. If you know what [the surgery] involves, then you know. If you don't, I won't tell you. I've got this phrase in my head that describes it. I can't say it—even now.'

Polly told me that she learned to fill in this silence, this inability to speak, with poetry. She bought a small notebook—small because it would be easier to hide. At first she would wait to get home after a shift to write down a few ideas, sometimes writing a whole poem in one evening. Later she would start writing on her bus journey home in the rain. Then she found that the need to put down words grew more urgent and she would scribble notes during handover and, eventually, would take herself to a corner of the ward, or even to storerooms or the toilets, to complete a short poem. She told me she found an outlet for her work in one of the online websites for nurse poets and, during her last years of working as a nurse, she spent many nights on the Caring Words website hosted at Manchester Metropolitan University (http://www.caringwords.mmu.ac.uk/). She has given permission for some of her first poems to appear in this book for the first time.

## You and me

> Sitting on a bus
> Thinking about us
> Windows streaming rain
> Thinking about your pain
> I can't forget
> How we met
> The hour before your death
> Brought out my best

It seemed to me that she found a kind of resilience in this practice. She said that the search for rhythms and rhymes reassured her that there was a structure somewhere during those times when she felt most in danger of being overwhelmed by nursing work. What is surprising is that, compared to other poetry written by nurses, her lines contain so few references to the actual work of nursing and only fleeting references to patients. My own research on resilience has suggested that nurses, and others, who have a confident understanding of the political structures that underpin their work might be considered more resilient than those who don't. But for Polly the structures that she needed to keep herself together were the structures of language itself. This 'keeping together', however, came at an increasing cost to her professional life. Her 'disappearances' from the ward became more frequent and lengthy, and they did not go unnoticed. Twice, she told me, she was on the verge of failing placements during her training because of her erratic behaviour.

'It shocked me big time, the second time. I literally had no idea how long I had been off with the muses. I actually tore my stuff up and told myself "this is crazy, this has got to stop". I didn't know at the time that this was actually my lifeline.'

Polly qualified as an adult nurse in 2010. She appreciated the independence that qualification brought:

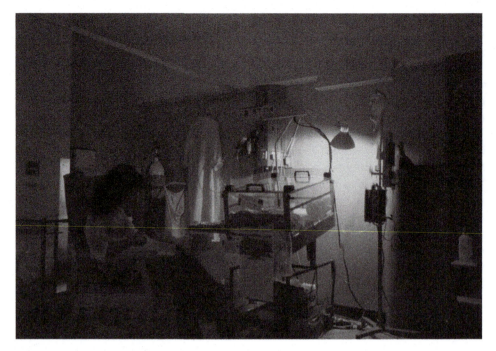

**FIGURE 7.1** The nightshift

'I think to be more independent as a nurse—because we used to be observed all the time and we couldn't be independently looking after patients; there was always somebody supervising us—I think we definitely needed it, I did. But if you're a qualified nurse, you are independently looking after patients and, you know, I think, you get the appreciation for that, you know, that I did something really good and I'm good, was good, at my job.'

From Polly's narrative, I got the impression that her first years of qualification went without incident. But it was three years later, in 2013, that Polly experienced what she described as a 'frightening relapse of poetic feeling'. I asked if she could remember what had occurred just before the 'relapse' but she told me that she could not. It had involved a considerable withdrawal from duty during a busy morning shift on a general surgical ward. Staff were sent to search for her and she was eventually found on a bench in the hospital foyer, her legs drawn up underneath her and hunched over an A4 pad that she had just taken from the hospital newsagent. She could still recite to me the lines of a short poem that she had started writing then.

## Falling

> We are all falling as snow
> Witnessed at night, in beauty and in blame
> We are all failing, fingers across the keys
> Extinguish the last flame

Her absence, of course, did not go down well and was reported upwards through various management levels; eventually, the decision was made for disciplinary action.

'They told me that I was being reported to the NMC and not to come in. I had to give up my name badge. I spent the next few weeks taking long walks in the park. I got a sick note and then basically left.'

Though the NMC decided that her case did not merit further action, Polly, like so many nurses whose reputation and fitness to practice has been questioned, resigned and did not return to nursing (see Chapter 8 for a similar verdict and outcome). Polly told me that she started voluntary work for a mental health charity and now helps to run workshops that encourage individuals in distress to write about their thoughts. I believe that she is relatively happy in this line of work, and it seems to suit her, but when I asked whether she still wrote poetry she did not give me an answer.

Does she have regrets?

'My path through life has been indirect—that's all. My friends and family were always puzzled that I could never answer their questions about how was my day at work [as a nurse]. I literally could not speak. But I noticed that as soon as I had a pen or pencil in my hand I could make something of what was happening, instead of events making something of me.'

Polly's realisations, gained at considerable personal and professional cost, reminded me of blogger Madeleine Mysko's not unpoetic conjectures about the way that nurses can approach writing poetry:

> [Nurses] are present at moments of human vulnerability. At the same time, the work that nurses do—often so close to our pain as to breathe the very air of it—demands a

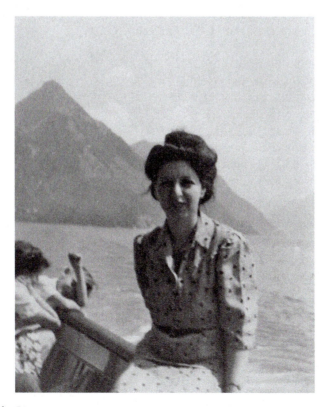

**FIGURE 7.2** Lake Lucerne

discipline that limits access to emotion. Good nurses keep a check on the feelings—fear, revulsion, anger, grief—that might compromise what they have to offer as professionals… The nurse [poet]'s approach might be described as professional barriers to emotion dismantled out of poetic necessity.

*http://www.rattle.com/when-the-poet-happens-to-be-a-nurse-by-madeleine-mysko/*

It was only the rigorous inquiry and the constraints of structure required by serious writing that allowed Polly to confront and make sense of her experiences as a nurse and then, I think, to move away from it. I know little about the world of poetry but I use the word 'serious' because I sense a difference between the few poems of Polly's that I have seen and the products of other sometimes well-known nurse poets who seem to wear their hearts on their sleeves.

Polly sent me, in the post, a photograph taken on a holiday she took with her aunt and a niece and nephew. She says it was taken on Lake Lucerne in Switzerland.

I want to end this chapter with one of the pieces she wrote during her last weeks of nursing, two reflections on empathy. She asks that it see the light of day in the pages of this book on resilience.

## Specialing Pena-Shokeir 2 syndrome / Nightshift in the hospital / A nurse's empathy

You down there are weeks old
You will not have a birthday party
No cake with a single flickering flame for you
No happy birthday to you
Different candles for you, I'm afraid
I up here, looking after your monitor
Flick her, they told me, when it falls down to 30
On my lap a comedy
I even laugh aloud
I flick you. You will die another time or another shift
I am alone in this angle-poise room with you
I will do my best for you

## Nightshift / A mother's empathy

Our hearts beat in parallel
Two millimetres apart
Yours tiny, mine large and bruised by you
Your heart against my heart
Flesh of my flesh
Your life soft and brief
Meat of my meat
Grief of my grief
A hospital light harrowing

White the cot's shroud
Our fevered hearts in parallel
Beat unavowed
Some say she breathes
Some say not
You die, I will die
As you rise up
So rise I

# 8

# SIMONE, THE NURSE WHO STOOD IN SOLIDARITY

## Working on the border between religion, madness and profession

We stand beside you in solidarity

This is the story of a community psychiatric nurse who works in a crisis team in a highly diverse area of south London. She tells how she approaches working alongside the religious faith of some of the clients. The team's challenge is sometimes to untangle psychosis and delusional beliefs from the teachings of various non-mainstream religious groups. She talks of working with local faith leaders and of 'standing beside clients in solidarity' as they pray to deities that she herself may not believe in.

I met Simone at F. Mondays on Brixton Hill in south London, close to the area that she works in. It was late spring when we met for the first time, just warm enough to sit outside in the café's lush back garden, away from the noise and business of the street and the constant interruption of emergency vehicle sirens. The second and last time that we met was on an unseasonably wet morning in the middle of summer and we sat at a small table next to a spikey cactus. Working in a community mental health crisis team has got to be one of the more unpredictable ways of earning a living in nursing, though also one that can be highly rewarding.

Brixton is still one of the more culturally diverse areas of London, despite the sometimes controversial gentrification that has transformed the area since the 1990s. In the 1950s and 1960s, it was one of the few parts of the capital that recent migrants from the West Indies were able to settle in. The sometimes bleak and windswept Windrush Square was given its present name in 1998 to mark the arrival of the *Empire Windrush* 50 years earlier in 1948; this boat brought 500 settlers from Jamaica to London, in response to recruitment drives intended to meet employment shortages in state-run services like the NHS and London Transport. Some say that the arrival of this boat in Tilbury Docks in June of that year marked the beginning of modern British multicultural society. The widespread prejudice of those days made it hard for Caribbean settlers to get a job, find accommodation and even open a bank account. In the 1980s, during Margaret Thatcher's office, there were riots in Brixton and major conflict in response to what was considered by many a racist and oppressive police force and, specifically, as a reaction to the 'sus law', allowing police to stop and search anyone they suspected of possible wrongdoing—in effect, mainly young black men. It has been a centre for reggae and

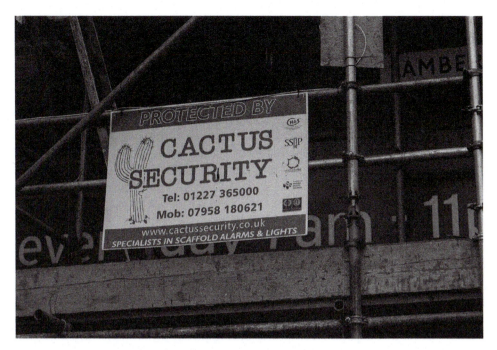

**FIGURE 8.1** Cactus Security sign in Brixton

Rastafari,[1,2] as well as an array of what I can best describe as non-mainstream religious groups. Some of these groups meet in unusual and sometimes hard to find rooms and buildings, such as the former industrial buildings at Copeland Park industrial estate in Peckham, fifteen minutes away on the 37.[3] This brief background sets the scene for the story that Simone told me about her work.

Her phrase that had me scrabbling for my pencil and pad at the start of our first meeting was 'We stand beside you in solidarity'. I could see that Simone was proud to be able to describe her work with clients in this way, although I sensed that her story was not going to be straightforward and that she was setting the context in order to bring up something that was troubling her. She had worked in south London as a mental health nurse for fifteen years, the last five as a member of a community crisis team. For many of her and her team's clients, religious and spiritual faith and beliefs play an influential, if not central, role in their lives. Her

---

1 According to the newspaper *The Voice* (www.voice-online.co.uk/article/sharing-emergence-rastafari-movement-britain), "The post-Windrush second generation found themselves feeling displaced and alienated from mainstream British society, and drew inspiration from the philosophies of black pride and identity cemented in the foundation of the Rastafari beliefs. The new-found identity was fluid, organic and connected them to their Caribbean and African heritage." The Rastafari HQ was sited in St. Agnes Place in nearby Kennington, SE11, for thirty years.

2 See also Henry (2012), who argues that reggae music and Rastafari created an arena for resistance and identity formation among African Caribbean communities in the UK in the 1980s.

3 A branch of the Cherubim & Seraphim Church has a room here. It is easy to assume that the use of previous commercial, sometimes decrepit and often ugly premises is simply to do with lack of funds, but it gives a strong message about the spirituality of these groups. The real action is happening on a spiritual realm, between the individual and God, perhaps mediated by the pastor or elder.

team's involvement in religion can take two forms. 'Sometimes the faith can be on the side of the loved ones—often it's the parents of one of our clients who are really distressed about their son or daughter—and sometimes those clients themselves can hold, or at least talk about holding, particular religious beliefs.'

'Our clients and their families want us to take their faith seriously and to build it into the way that we care for them. Even NHS policy says that services should provide spiritual support for patients and relatives—and staff—with chaplains and other faith representatives, but the reality is that we still basically treat people with medication. If anything, our ears prick up when clients talk about religious experiences or beliefs. It is hard sometimes not to see it as evidence of their condition.'

I asked Simone what she meant by 'spiritual', 'religious' and 'faith' because, although textbooks give distinct definitions of these terms, I was interested in how someone with such a strong involvement in the lives of people with mental health problems understood to what extent these concepts might overlap in practice.

'Everybody asks that—and can you be spiritual without being religious or religious without being spiritual? I think everybody is spiritual—when they are deeply moved by a piece of music or by a sudden stillness in nature, touched by a sudden strangeness, an unexpected reversal in life, a sense of something beyond.'

'Transcendent?'

'Yes. And religion happens when people get together to formalise this and fix it in a system of beliefs. When you can say that you believe them all, all of the beliefs, then you can say you are a member of that religion. And religions have practices. Some you can do alone, but mostly they harness the power of coming together. A hundred people saying a prayer out loud together is very different to saying it in your own head in your bedroom. The same with singing or dancing. Something special is happening.'

'What about faith?'

'Well, faith, belief. That's why we are talking, isn't it?'

Simone had contacted me to talk about the dilemmas of working with clients who had mental health problems, a diagnosis of schizophrenia perhaps, who were also members of religious groups, some of which have strange, or rather, unfamiliar beliefs or practices.

'Some people say a belief is something that you are persuaded of. It might be because you have some kind of proof, something rational, or it might be more abstract—"I believe that bad people will eventually get their just deserts" or "I believe that Jesus died to pay for my sins and that He will come to judge us at the end of the world". But beliefs don't necessarily need proof. Having confidence in these beliefs and acting on them, making them part of your life, I would call faith.'

'So what is a delusion? How do you know the difference between a religious belief and a delusion?'

'Well, the kind of distinguishing principle that you often read is that, while 'faith' inevitably has some questioning built into it, delusions are characterised by certainty; or others say that religious faith beliefs are shared by a community, delusions are more individual. But what's confusing is that delusions often have religious content—"I've been called by God to do some particular task".[4] And then, how do we know how shared a belief is? When a client with schizophrenia tells us that he is expecting the Second Coming at any moment, or something more

---

4 This is one definition from psychologists (Iyassu, Jolley et al. 2014): Delusions are a cardinal feature of psychotic illness, present in around three quarters of people with a schizophrenia spectrum diagnosis. Religious themes are

bizarre, we sometimes try to contact a local faith leader and ask them—is this something you really teach?[5] Often that is really helpful and gives us confidence in dealing with that client.'

'So someone with faith is likely to be racked by doubts. That's certainly the theme of books and films…'[6]

'But that's not always true. I know quite a few people of faith who have unquestioning certainty about their beliefs, but they are not schizophrenic as far as I know. I think it is something more about psychic structure: some people fill life's enigmas with a certainty. They seem certain about everything, often that their misfortunates are other people's faults—but that's another question. Others are more neurotic and are always questioning themselves.'

'What about these so-called anomalous experiences? For example voices, visions and demons? Do you think that religions encourage these kinds of experiences and beliefs? Some say that religions foster psychotic episodes.'

'The short answers are, yes to the first part of the question—many religions do indeed talk about voices, visions and beliefs in malign spiritual forces—but no to the second question—I don't think that religion fosters psychotic illness. What's true is that, when clients talk about voices, visions and other exotic religious experiences and beliefs, this can lead professionals to the mistaken belief that a person is suffering from psychosis when they are not.'

'So how do you work with clients, and their families, who have particular religious beliefs but you don't share them?'

'That is a good question and, in a way, that's why I contacted you. About a year ago we started working with Ojanomare. He's a guy born in Nigeria but who lived and studied in London for most of his life. The name means "I have met the challenge". He was, and still is, a member of a West African church that meets not too far from here. Ojan got into some conflict with a relative, a cousin I think, over inheritance of some land. And this cousin practised magic, even though this is forbidden in his branch of faith, and, during an argument, this cousin put a curse on Ojanomare, telling him he would die. OK, so Ojan stopped eating and drinking. He became completely withdrawn and would not leave his room. Ojan's parents were beside themselves and called in a doctor, and he was eventually admitted to hospital where he was started on IV fluids and was also diagnosed with schizophrenia on the grounds that his belief about being cursed was a delusion and was threatening his health. That's when we are called in. Ojanomare continued to believe he had been cursed and got worse. There was even the fear that he would die. At that point, his parents contacted another magician—I don't know how you find a magician—who, I don't know how or what he did, was able to remove the curse from Ojan. After this, Ojan began to eat and drink and his mood improved quickly. He was discharged two days later. Everyone was relieved and happy.'

'So was that some kind of shared delusion or was he really cursed?'

---

common across delusion categories and types, with between a fifth and two-thirds of all delusions reflecting religious content. To be classified as a religious delusion, the belief must be idiosyncratic, rather than accepted within a particular culture or subculture.

5 The text concerned with the diagnosis of delusional disorder in the Diagnostic and Statistical Manual of Mental Disorders indicates that 'an individual's cultural and religious background must be taken into account in evaluating the possible presence of delusional disorder'( Holoyda and Newman 2016). It is unclear to what degree 'cultural and religious background' could include participation in a cult. Holoyda and Newman's paper provides an in-depth discussion of cults and shared delusions in extreme cases.

6 I am thinking of Alfred Hitchcock's *I Confess* (1953), Ingmar Bergman's *Winter Light* (1963), Brendan Gleeson in John Michael McDonagh's *Calvary* (2014) and more recently Ethan Hawke's stunning portrayal of priest Ernst Toller in Paul Schrader's 2018 *First Reformed*.

'That's not why I brought this up. While Ojanomare was ill, and everyone expected him to die, his parents prayed for him. And the opportunity came for my colleague Martin and myself to pray with them in the hospital. I started by saying that our approach is to stand beside you in solidarity. Though we don't necessarily share your faith, we support you in expressing your deepest wishes, in this case for their son to live. Sometimes we literally stand shoulder to shoulder with those who pray. It's a keystone of the way we work and it gives us a huge amount of satisfaction. It gives us a real sense of closeness to our clients and their families and makes us feel we are making a difference.'

'Supporting families.'

'Well, it's always felt like much more than supporting. When someone is praying, often they are desperate and it can be very special to share that, very moving, one of those moments when you feel glad to be a nurse. It is right at the heart of our motivation as professionals but also as people too. Well, about six months after this crisis, Ojan and his parents came in for a clinic follow-up. Everything was resolved and there were no problems. Everything was fine. After the appointment, I was in the waiting room checking something with another client, speaking quietly, and they, Ojan and his parents, were also sitting in the waiting room with their backs to me, chatting to another of our clients.'

'They didn't know that you were there.'

'No, they had no idea I was there. But obviously, I could hear everything that they were saying. Ojan's father was talking to the sister of one of our clients with schizophrenia, someone who is completely devoted to advocating for her brother, not from the same part of the world as Ojan's parents but also someone who is very religious. She's an active member of her mosque. We had many conversations about her faith, I remember, and how it gave her hope and strength to stick with her brother through some quite scary times. He, Ojan's father, asked her about what she thought of our team and she replied that we were good with the technical things but the stuff about standing in solidarity and praying with her, she did not believe. She said that we were being very professional, but she knew that we did not share her beliefs and that it was obvious to her and that it was actually quite embarrassing for her. Ojanomare's father basically agreed with her. He said that he wished we had not done that.'

'So what did you think about that?'

'I was frozen. It was the last thing I expected to hear. I've had time to reflect on it now. It was as if the version of myself that I had built up over many years was stripped away, just by that short exchange. I actually felt different in my body. I did not feel like me. That is what it felt like at the time. I had this sudden insight that other people weren't seeing me in the way that I hoped and assumed they did. I wondered if I had been living out my own delusion for most of my professional life.'

'By your earlier distinction between a delusion and a faith, this sounds more like a faith.'

'It's shared by many.'

'Yes.'

'So I basically, after that event and ruminating on it, I realised that it would be impossible to carry on as before. I started reading about resilience. Everyone was talking about it. I did gratefulness training. I realised though that, instead of carrying on with my delusion, and propping it up, I needed to understand something about the profession as a whole and my part in it. I realised that the world would not fall apart if I started questioning some of my profession's cherished beliefs.'

We ordered more coffee. One of the baristas told us joyfully that, on her first day at work there, she had dropped a cup, a teapot and finally a saucepan of hot milk.

Simone continued. 'I remember vividly. I went to an RCN Congress quite a few years back. I had never been to one before. A mental health nurse was giving an impassioned talk. I think it was a debate about the government not valuing the profession—a recurrent theme. He was talking about the personal satisfaction he got from giving meticulous care to a man with Alzheimer's, taking immense trouble and time to feed him a meal and making a real difference to his quality of life. He was saying that his sense of satisfaction, of making a difference was proof of the value of his work with that man, his work as a whole and proof of the value of the profession. He got rapturous applause. You could imagine we were at a religious event. I thought this was a great statement. It was very moving, the whole event was, full of confessions and tears. Looking back now, today, I am a little sceptical.'

'On what grounds? It's not unusual to hear this.'

'Because, I think that nurse who spoke is mixing up the satisfying of his own needs with meeting the needs of clients and patients. Just because he walks away from an encounter with a patient or client feeling glowing is no measure or guarantee that anyone he is looking after is feeling the same. I think he is making a big mistake.'

'But everyone applauded. How many nurses attend these events?'

'Thousands. That's what makes it a faith. So for me, I think that the idea of standing in solidarity alongside others who believe did work for *me*. I enjoyed saying it each time I said it.'[7]

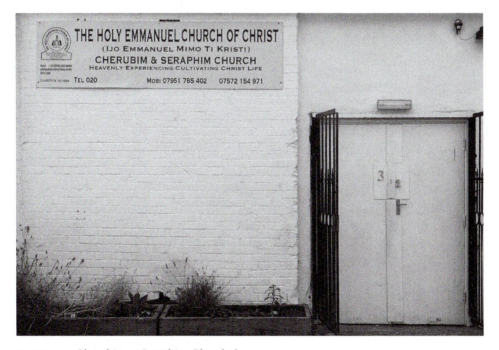

**FIGURE 8.2** Cherubim & Seraphim Church door

7 Simone pointed me toward this quotation from a paper she had read: 'For some the formation of delusions is adaptive in combatting purposelessness and hopelessness and provides a new sense of identity and a change from fear, worry, depression and boredom towards feeling lively, enthusiastic, interested and peaceful" (Simms, 2012, p. 4).

'Yes, it is a powerful statement. I remember wanting to note it down when we first met. So don't you say it any more? Don't you do it any more?'

'No. I don't say it any more. Actually, I've learned to listen. I thought I was being good at listening, but now I say less and I watch what happens, or what I think is happening. When I am with clients and their families, I ask more questions. Actually, I am very interested in comparative religion. Did you know that Rastafari describes itself as the religion of oppressed people all over the world?'

After our meeting, I decided to find my way to Copeland Park. I remember that it was still raining heavily and that the collapsible umbrella I had with me more or less collapsed. Even in the rain, it was a relief to discard it in a bin and leave it behind. I caught the 37 bus to Peckham Rye, travelling in my favourite seat up at the top in the front through affluent Dulwich before getting off near the industrial estate and walking down there in the now easing rain. The estate is full of cafes and community projects today but there is still some evidence of religious meetings. As well as the Cherubim and Seraphim Church, there are the Gospel Auditorium and the World Outreach Evangelistic Ministries. After making a way through the sometimes narrow, dark and puddle-filled passages between buildings, twisting unpredictably, you take a sudden turning and find yourself on bright, busy and bustling Rye Lane.

# 9

# JOHN, THE TRAUMA NURSE

One of the many possible titles that I discussed with the publishers of this book included the phrase 'nursing on the frontline'. Although partly problematic because the term has become overused, I imagined that if ideas of resilience would be thought about anywhere it would be in areas of nursing where practitioners deal with extreme trauma. I was particularly interested in whether there was a realisation within such services of the need to develop built-in organisational resilience.

I set about searching for a contact with whom I could discuss different flavours of resilience in this kind of extreme setting and who could possibly provide some material for this book. A chain of recommendations, phone calls, dead-ends and fortuitous meetings later, I found myself in John's office on the edge of a wet industrial estate in southwest London, next to an ambulance station that was in the process of being demolished. Rain seems to have followed me around during the preparation for this book and I had to step over large puddles to enter the building where he works. John is a senior trauma nurse with a special interest in resilience. I learned that what I just described as his interest had a deeply personal origin in dealing with his own trauma. Despite his work in the area, it was his personal accounts that I found most captivating in terms of my own investigations into the varied way that people use the term resilience and search for, and appear to find, solutions to the human problem of adversity. This was one of the last interviews I conducted for this book and I was beginning to realise that, along with ways to keep dry, it was responses to trauma in and around nursing work that most interested me.

But first, what is trauma nursing? Some definitions distinguish between Emergency Department (ED) nursing and trauma nursing. In some settings, the trauma centre is where patients arrive when they are, to use one phrase I encountered, 'beyond ill'. But many accounts do not differentiate the two. These seriously ill patients may have been brought to the ED after a car crash, a major sporting accident, a stab wound, a gunshot or some other serious injury that requires urgent medical attention. Other trauma nurses may work on the scene of such events. Discussing the abilities needed by nurses in this area, one website says 'Trauma nurses must be able to act quickly to save a life hanging in the balance. They must remain calm under extreme pressure, be strong in the face of catastrophic injuries, manage multiple priorities and

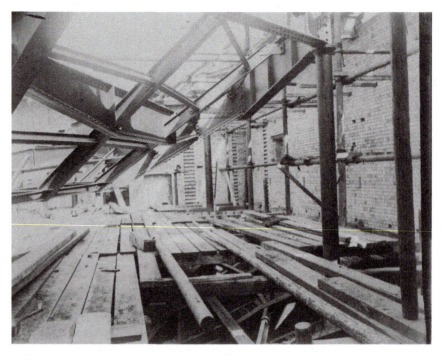

**FIGURE 9.1** Demolition of the ambulance station

tasks, and quickly provide and follow instructions in chaotic situations' (https://nurse.org/resources/trauma-nurse/). That appears to be quite an ask but, as Daniel Chambliss says, nurses can be good at 'routinising the traumatic' in ways essential to get the job done but which may turn out to be less helpful in the long term (Chambliss 1996).

John had recently—the day before we met—returned from a trip training nurses and medics in the effects of exposure to traumatic work and he looked tired. John is in early middle age with a face that you could describe as weathered. Without invitation from me, he began by telling me his thoughts about resilience. It was not until about twenty minutes into our interview that I was able to get out my notebook and start to work through the few questions that I had prepared.

One of his colleague's responses to dealing with trauma had clearly made an impression on him and he returned to it more than once:

'Resilience is interesting. A lot of my team have been exposed to levels of trauma, as you can imagine. Some deal with it really well—and I was having a chat to one of my team recently. He's thoroughly pragmatic. It's a door that's closed. "I did the best I could do and I moved on." And he doesn't, it seems at the moment, really re-live any of what he went through. He's just closed the door. He has, I think you'd say, stone-walled going back there. But other people struggle with the fact that they have guilt, for example: "Did I get there quickly enough? Did I do enough? Could I have done more? Could I have saved that person?" The point is they can't change it. Some people are just not able to move on from that.'

He went on to talk about some ideas for a strategy that might prevent the development of post-traumatic stress disorder (PTSD), based on his own private concerns about resilience.

'I have wondered, from my perspective, if I, personally, would find it helpful, cathartic,[1] to write down my own experiences, at a major incident, say. Anonymised, fictionalised even…'

'Fictionalised?'

'Yes, why not? Powerful points are no less true when they're a result of a kind of flight of imagination.'

'What do you mean?'

'I could write down what I was exposed to and work out for myself what really stressed me, but the "I" might be a persona I develop to give me a freedom to explore and extend possible responses. And therefore somebody else reading that after the event would maybe be able to say, "Well, this is how that person felt after the event. This is what made them worry or, more importantly, this is what they did about it. And if *they* now feel OK, then I will be OK." So I suppose if people enter, at the level of emotion, into my scenarios they may already be prepared to deal with and think about those issues when they encounter such an event in real life, if you like.'

'Like an emotional inoculation?'

'Exactly.'

One of the many definitions of trauma is an event or events that cannot be put into language by the person who experiences them. I will speak about this later. I see John's proposal as an attempt to make it more acceptable to speak about highly stressful events along with describing some practical steps that the person who experienced these took.[2] John applied that approach to his work with other nurses working in his field.

'So I ran, for a while, a small group made up of nurses who'd witnessed trauma—of all kinds—and at one point I asked them: "Is this the first time that you have talked about this?" And all of them said, "Yes, this is the first time we have actually sat down and felt we could be supported in being able to talk to anyone about our experiences." They had found it cathartic, but when I asked them what model we could use in the NHS to help people like them, none of them had any idea. I was quite shocked. But I asked them to write down a story, as I said just now, either just for themselves or to share anonymously on our Intranet to start a support network. But it died a death. It just didn't happen and I haven't been able to get to the bottom of why it didn't happen.'

Nevertheless, John is convinced that a simple way of sharing experiences could be beneficial and avoid subsequent problems:

'I've spoken to people that are struggling with things now, sometimes years after the traumatic event, they're now struggling with PTSD symptoms. So the most resilient-appearing people—because you look at some people and you think, "Nothing's ever going to break you." And it's the people that we least expect to break that are… It's just getting through to people that they can access support when they need it.'

I asked whether recruitment to this kind of service has the effect of selecting nurses who are likely to have the kind of resilience that people talk about.

---

1 What is catharsis? The word is used freely. It comes from Greek. As a medical term it means to cleanse or purge the body of unwanted material. However, Greek philosopher Aristotle used the term in *The Poetics*, a book primarily about drama, to describe a purging of the pre-existing strong emotions of an audience that is effected by involvement in a tragedy, where the emotions of *terror*, evoked by seeing a character suffering frightening misfortune, and *pity*, a kind of identification with that character, are finely balanced.

2 I have slipped from using the word 'trauma' to the common psychological term 'stress', partly because John goes on to reach for a psychological term himself and partly for other reasons that I will talk about later.

John acknowledged that this was the big question.

'I was speaking to my colleague who has got this very pragmatic "No, I'm not going to go back and revisit some of my experiences. I don't want to, and I think I did the best job I could, and there's no point in dwelling over it because I'm not going to change the outcome. People died and actually there's no way we could have saved them. Their injuries were incompatible with life. They died and that was the best thing for them. They wouldn't have had quality of life." And he's compartmentalised that. He's very logical about it. He's justified it and he hasn't broken. As I said to you, other people aren't able to have such a knife through that coping mechanism. But what happens sometimes is that life gets in the way of someone's professional resilience. Someone that's dealt with an emergency, they've dealt with the trauma of all of that, that they have done as good a job as they possibly could, and then in their personal life a parent may die suddenly. And their world implodes.'

'So how does that work?'

'I think you feel very vulnerable. You feel that you are out of control. Maybe. I'm just repeating what I've been told. Or sometimes people have no choice. Sometimes they are taken back there because they start to dream it. We've got no control over what we dream, have we, and then it takes you back.'

John then told me about his involvement in a specific high-profile major emergency in the capital. For reasons of confidentiality, I am not identifying the event. John had a prolonged involvement and spoke about the effect it had on him.

'Certainly when I came back after about 48 hours, not constant, but heavy involvement, when I came home, I didn't realise I was stressed. I didn't realise I was stressed at all. I didn't think I'd changed. I didn't think I was any different… [Details about where and for how long]… I was lucky I was able to speak to my partner who also works in healthcare. And that also made me think that I had told him things that I hadn't. So, that only became apparent when I went to see, as part of post-event stress management, I went see a counsellor, well, she's a manager for another team, someone who has got vast experience and that we don't necessarily work with. So its speaking to somebody in a non-judgemental way. And it's a twenty-minute interview, or should be, and three hours later I was still in there. And, ah,[3] I have no idea where any of that came from. I just talked and she let me talk. I went home that evening and I felt such a relief. I hadn't realised that I was hanging on to certain things that I'd witnessed and wondered about.'

'So you were able to speak and that speaking about it was enough to…'

'Yes. And I think that sometimes that is enough. That was the first opportunity to debrief and to go through it, and then she started to ask me questions such as "well why do you feel that way?" And then I was able to actively reflect with her and came up with certain conclusions, and then I went home that evening and I felt as if the weight of the world had been lifted off my shoulders. And I started to speak to my partner about certain things and he said, "You never told me that". "Of course I have. I told you about it when I got back." "No, no, that's the first time I've ever heard that." So then we were able to start talking and it just opens the door. It gives you permission to start talking about these things, and then we got closer, not that we had drifted apart, however, we then felt closer because we were sharing things that were important to us, and I think if I hadn't had that opportunity to speak then I

---

3 I did not know how to transcribe the sound that John made here. It was a cross between a heavy exhalation and a muted cry of pain. I imagined the memory was clearly still vivid for him.

probably would have still been hanging on to certain things. My partner said, "You went away from me but not all of you came back…" 'You change. Events change you.'

'Forever? '

'Well, not necessarily because I, once I started to talk and once I started to deal with what I hadn't even perceived as an issue, life got back to normal and then my partner objectively was able to say, "You're back", because you know, you've brought back your personality. He said, "You were subdued." And I couldn't believe it. I was asking, "How was I different?" "You were a little bit subdued, you didn't really want to do anything." He said, "Your spark wasn't there." He said, "that's the bit you left behind and suddenly, once you'd had that opportunity to talk, you were suddenly a different—you were back to yourself again."'

'So that was that?'

'Yes, you don't even see it yourself. I just didn't see it. I didn't see I was being, ah, so distant I suppose. I remember working with someone once who just didn't realise she was so affected, she was the manager, and it was everybody else's problem. I remember that service. People were covered in eczema, they were so stressed. That's why I left and now work in a team where the managers acknowledge that support and counselling is an absolute priority. If I hadn't made this move I would be—I don't know. Back then I felt that I had no value, that I was just a functioning non-human unit that had no requirement to be cared about and I don't think it's changed that much in the years that I've been away. Maybe there are good pockets of support for nurses. I don't know.'

Two words that John used caught my attention. He described how the impact on individuals of what resilience researchers referred to as adversity could result in these individuals 'breaking'.

The other word, used from time to time in resilience research, and used many times during our conversation, was trauma. As with many often used words, familiarity can cover over a variation in meaning and intention. First, I asked John what he meant when he talked about 'resilience' to 'trauma'.

'It's coping with, dealing with, reactions at the time and those visual images, being able to compartmentalise those.'

'Compartmentalise?'

'As in, put it into a box, into a logical sequence of events…'

'Another word you've used is "broken"…'

'Yes.'

'Or "break". What do you mean by that?'

'If you break, you lose your ability to deal with life. You go back to those times when—well, it comes back to control, to feeling vulnerable. Some people can't get out of bed. They can't function. They feel so—depressed is the wrong word—so physically low and often that's down to guilt, it's down to losing that sense of belonging in their own mind. A lack of value, of being valued. The fact that they didn't do enough so therefore they're to blame for somebody's death in some way. Sometimes people are very emotional and they will cry all the time.'

'Using this work "break", it sounds a sudden, dramatic thing. It reminds me of spy stories about the man that wouldn't break under interrogation.'

'No, not necessarily. I think there are lots of symptoms that people ignore. An example I gave you earlier was where I didn't know I was behaving in a different way until something happened that made me realise I was different. Had my partner not said those words and I hadn't realised, I may well have been broken. I would then have carried on this being different, being angry, whatever my symptoms were, to the point where I physically couldn't function. And that's the difference between those that develop PTSD and those that don't. And I don't know what makes you able to not break—some of it comes down to whether you're dealt a hard blow in your life.'

At this point, my recording was interrupted by John's administrator who knocked on his office door and asked us if we wanted more tea. I looked at my watch and realised that we had been talking for an hour, and I wondered whether she is briefed to interrupt meetings that look as though they are overrunning. It was time to draw to a close, but I had one final question.

I asked John what had taken him into this field of work.

'In conventional services, critical care was as far as I was able to go, before joining this team, because I am not able to dehumanise, to separate the human element from the technical. I can't disassociate the two. Even before I moved into this area, I would put myself in the position of the—I remember I was sitting by the bed and I couldn't—that's when I had to walk away because I couldn't escape from the emotion of the job that I was doing.'

'What was that emotion? '

'Grief. Grief and loss. I would sit there as if that were my father's hand I was holding. And that's when you know you can't leave it behind at the bedside.'

John then told me the story of the death of his father. At times I felt that this was still a raw emotion for him, but then he would shift to describing the events and his response to them in a way that appeared to be saying that everything was sorted, or compartmentalised, to take up a word that John used.

'As I say, there's lots of things that happen to you in your life. I lost my father when I was twenty. I barely knew him. He was the classic absent father. Never there, certainly never there for me. I never got a sense he valued me. And when he was there he was distant, silent. Not exactly violent but arbitrary and tyrannical, I suppose. You never knew what was going to happen next. It made it hard even to make simple plans, say about going out with friends. I ought to have been relieved when he died but I'm sure, looking back, that I was in a deep depression for quite some time as I came through the grieving process that I hear people describing, the different stages. I've read about them. And then suddenly I realised, well, there *is* a point to life because— what happened shortly after his death, I went travelling and I went to India—I didn't go to find myself of course, it was just an opportunity to get some exercise. And I visited Varanasi. Hindus go on pilgrimage there to bathe in the Ganges, but also the same sacred river is used for funerals, for cremations. Hundreds of bodies are burned there every day, in plain sight. People believe that if the dead person's ashes are scattered on the Ganges at Varanasi they will finally escape the cycle of birth and death. Sometimes, I can tell you, there is a lot more than ashes left when the bodies are set afloat on the river. The guy that was escorting us took us to see this. It was very confronting and the heat was almost unbearable, the heat from the flames. Between the chiming of bells I could hear the bodies hissing in the flames. Some actually sat up. And I found myself getting very, very emotional. Our guide looked at me as though I was strange. "Why are you crying? Why are you upset?" I remember I was sweating and my hair was covered in ash. I said, "I don't understand. There's somebody who's died down there. And his family are sitting drinking tea and chatting like it's a nice day out. It doesn't make any sense." But he said it's a celebration. And how different to us. We grieve and mourn death—they celebrate life. And I felt suddenly very disconnected having been so sad for the loss of my dad. And then I felt foolish and selfish {laughs} about the way that I'd grieved for so long, and it just made me see things through a different lens and then I suddenly felt much better.'

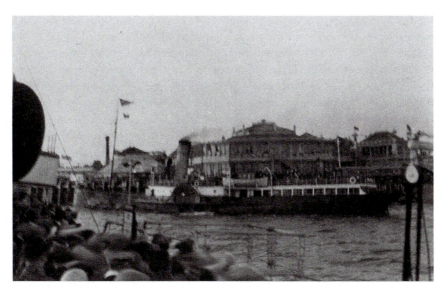

**FIGURE 9.2** A river crowd

I was interested in how John understood trauma because I had been reading, on my way to our meeting, some early definitions of the term by psychoanalysts. For Freud, trauma, and I think he is particularly thinking of childhood trauma, is something that cannot be processed by the conscious mind and, because of this, it continues to have an unconscious influence on the individual. Some say that this original trauma has a distinctly visual character. For Lacan,[4] trauma exists in 'the real', one of the three registers of human existence proposed by him, the others being the 'symbolic', which is broadly speaking the register of language, and the 'imaginary', the field of images and the imagination, characterised by illusion and alienation. The feature of the 'real' is that it cannot be put into language. The real, and trauma within it, will resist any attempt to do so. I wondered at the start of our conversation whether John was looking toward this when he spoke of trauma being that which individuals could not put into compartments or categories—language, of course, is above all a system of categories. But he went on to describe the resolution of two particularly difficult encounters for him. I think there is a difference between the not uncommon, in fact the now common-sense, notion that it is good to speak about problems, fears, etc. and psychoanalytic ideas about the nature and impact of trauma. From a psychoanalytic viewpoint, someone who has experienced trauma is unlikely to find a sudden resolution after a single encounter with a therapist. One commentator summarises one view of the impossibility of speaking directly about trauma:

> …the patient [person in psychoanalysis] can recollect his past minus the traumatic events. The traumatic events are unsymbolised for the subject; therefore, the subject cannot possibly recall those events; no matter how hard the subject might try, they would not overcome the void created by the trauma they have undergone.
>
> *Yansori 2018*

4 French psychoanalyst Jacques Lacan (1901–1981) combined Freud's ideas with the structuralist principles of Claude Levi-Strauss and others to develop a highly fertile, if complex, set of theories about the human psyche.

So I was left with a mystery, as we shook hands and I made my way down the stairs of John's building and across the still-wet car park. John seemed to have described to me events that could clearly be understood as traumatic: his 48 hours of dealing with a major event with many serious casualties and the immersive experience of cremation in Varanasi following the death of his father. Yet, for both occasions, John told of a sudden release from suffering. The first was as a result of a session with a counsellor and the second after an exchange with his travel guide and a sudden realisation that some cultures do not appear to grieve over death as he had done for his father. I also remembered his repeated reference to his colleague who was able to take what he described as a logical and compartmentalised approach to his witnessing of traumatic incidents. I was not sure whether John saw this as suspicious and possibly storing up trouble for the future or was acknowledging that this was simply one apparently effective approach.

As my exploration of resilience and how people talk about it and enact it was drawing to a close, I was beginning to be aware of one thing: the singularity of different people's responses to, or rather interactions with, adversity.

# 10

# MIRIAM'S STORY[1]

A patient in a hospital is dying. In front of him on an awkward hospital table, designed to fit, on shopping-trolley wheels, under a bed but in reality always getting in the way, is a bowl of soapy water. A nurse is attempting to shave him but his head keeps dropping forward, making her job difficult. She pushes his chin upwards with the side of her left hand and continues, with her free hand, to shave, holding a flimsy plastic razor that is not, and never would be, up to the job. It is awkward to shave someone like this. Curtains are drawn around the bed and there is little room, what with the table, the large plastic bowl of water, the clinging fabric of the curtain and now the drooping head, for manoeuvre. There are two other, more or less identical, beds in this small room that is situated to the left, when approached from the front, of the nurses' station. Nurses with even moderate experience of hospital organisation would know that patients whose beds are in these rooms—there is another room, a mirror image of this one to the right of the station—are there for a particular reason.

We are up on the ninth floor of a teaching hospital, the first parts of which were built in the 1970s. There are thirteen floors in total, excluding basements that house departments never seen by patients and rarely by the public. The windows up above ground level do not open but look out over the calm distance of a grassy hill bisected by a busy main road. We can see that, outside, heavy slow-moving cloud covers the entire sky. One recent Google review of the hospital observes 'Very good service, but quite a long wait time'. Another reads 'Shame, as it could be such an amazing place given enough staff'. Another notes, in a more neutral voice, that the hospital has a shopping centre, restaurants and children's play area.

---

1 The Foreword to my last book, on critical resilience, included mention of the story of Miriam, who was a fellow student nurse during my own training. Some readers found her story moving and I have included a more detailed account here, taken from my notes of recent conversations with others who knew her, have vivid memories of the events and are still in the profession. Thank you especially to J.L. and W.G. who drew my attention to some minor factual inaccuracies in the earlier account. I include the story here in order to show how easy it is to make mistakes when looking for resilience.

Miriam told us afterwards how irritated she was becoming with her patient that morning for being uncooperative. He was an elderly man, possibly in his eighties, with the bottoms of his pyjama trousers cut off hurriedly it seemed by the evidence of many lose threads, turning them, for a reason Miriam could not understand, into shorts, just above the knees. She continued to struggle.

'A staff nurse made a little slit opening in the curtains and peered over my shoulder, frowned slightly at Mr D, then came in, crouched down and took his hand to try to find a pulse', Miriam told us. 'And when she said, without turning to me, "I think he's gone", I remember not feeling much, just a little guilty at pushing him. Then I realised that there seemed to be no surprise that he had died. It was all very undramatic. It was my very first meeting with Mister Death.'

'The staff nurse told me to clear away the washing things and, when I got back, one of the doctors was there and confirmed he had passed away. We moved him into a position of repose and the staff nurse somehow produced a vase of bright yellow flowers and put them on the table—on the spot where the washing bowl had been only a few minutes before. It was then that I realised that Mr D's wife, also elderly, had been sitting outside the curtains all along. The staff nurse showed her in and she said thank you to all of us. I noticed then that half of Mr D's face was clean-shaven. Later that shift, the staff nurse took me aside, looked me in the eyes and asked if I was alright. I remember cheerily saying I was fine, because I was. It was not upsetting, it was just strange.'

Neither of my informants could remember whether this incident occurred during Miriam's first or second clinical placement but it was certainly early on in her training. I remember some of us talking quietly among ourselves about Miriam's ability to cope so calmly with her first death. We were extremely impressed, a little jealous, and we put it down to the fact that Miriam had come from a family of locally well-known nurses. She had nursing in her blood. On our first day of the course, she had told the class, with a huge amount of pride, that both her mother and grandmother were nurses. And, in fact, so was her aunt. I remember one tutor's sudden recognition, 'So *you* are the daughter of Vera [___].'

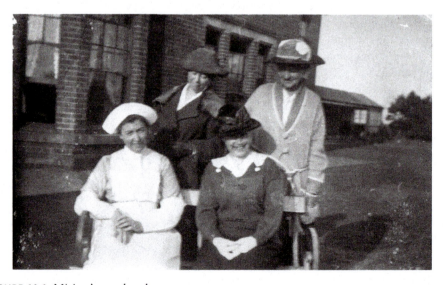

**FIGURE 10.1** Miriam's grandmother

At some point during the second year of our training, I remember the phrase 'Miriam has been dealt a difficult hand' being used. My informants could not tell me exactly the first time that this was said or whether we had started to use this phrase ourselves or had overheard some of our tutors' private concerns one day. Two of our tutors were twins—each other's twins.

It is difficult to tell the story of Miriam's misfortunes without the feeling that they are simply being listed to prove a point and to get to the end of her story. I have also thought many times that there is something unbelievable about this sequence of events. However, the chronology, if not every small detail, is corroborated by others who also witnessed them, albeit in a slightly oblique way. Miriam started Year Two of training with a placement in an Accident and Emergency (A&E) department. This was a prized placement as everyone wanted that kind of edgy experience but most ended up on orthopaedics, endlessly lifting frightened and heavily plastered patients off and onto bedpans. I privately wondered whether Miriam received preferential treatment because tutors were not a little in awe of her family and sensed her future potential. Not very long after her arrival in A&E, staff were signing out a dose of the painkiller Fentanyl and found that a capsule of this drug had already been signed out and no one remembered, so they said, doing this. After an investigation, they discovered a number of similar suspicious signings under fictitious patient names. The beginning of the incidents appeared to coincide with the start of Miriam's placement and, upon examination of the duty rota, it seemed that she was working on the ward during each of the occasions. In addition, her keenness, arriving early and staying late for shifts, was seen as evidence of possible 'diversion' of the department's drugs. Miriam was formally interviewed by the ward manager, a senior manager, the senior tutor and a representative from Human Relations. It was suggested to her that she had a secret drug addiction and, at one point, her room was searched. None of us, of course, knew what was happening at the time, though we sensed a strange atmosphere within the school and whenever her name was mentioned. We gradually began to understand the events a number of weeks later. Despite the strict confidentiality of the procedure, some nurses cannot resist telling a good story. It seemed that an inquiry finally proved that Miriam could not have been responsible for the thefts because the senior tutor gave assurances that Miriam was in the school for supervisions on many of the occasions when drugs had been fraudulently taken. It was also questioned whether Miriam as a student would have access, unaccompanied, to any drugs. The case was dropped.

What puzzled us most, once we began to piece this story together from unguarded statements and overheard talk, was that Miriam seemed her usual positive, well-presented self throughout the weeks of what must have been a traumatic ordeal. I am not sure if the true identity of the drug thief ever came to light. Miriam never revealed that this had happened and, though a few of us were aware of it, we also made sure that we did not ever bring it up.

Nearly everyone looked forward to community placements. It is a chance to get away from the hierarchical atmosphere of the hospital and work and learn in a more relaxed and autonomous setting. It can be an eye-opener to see how people live in their own homes and it is fun to be driven around pretty villages, as most of us were, by Community Nurses. It was driving, however, that set the stage for the next event that contributed to the adversity that Miriam experienced. On the way to visit a patient, with Miriam travelling as the passenger, the Community Nurse's car was hit in the rear by a Luton lorry, a medium to large size truck. She was waiting at a junction to turn right when the lorry swerved from a corner behind her. It struck a number of parked cars before ploughing into the back of the nurse's car. Both Miriam and the Community Nurse, who was also her mentor, appeared unhurt after the accident, but her mentor began to suffer from the effect of whiplash injuries over the following week and was sent home from work. She was, we were shocked to hear, never able to work again. We also read in the local newspaper that, though the lorry driver was charged with driving under the influence and received a driving ban, the insurers refused to accept that the nurse's injuries meant she was unable to work and this resulted in a lengthy court case during which Miriam was called as a witness. The nurse was successful and received compensation for lost earnings, though she was devastated to lose the only career she had ever wanted, we read in the article, since the age of four.

As I started to say earlier, none of these misfortunes are uncommon; yet, it is hard to do justice to the reality of the series of blows that life dealt Miriam during this period. At Easter of Year Two, Miriam was granted compassionate leave. Her mother had been taken ill and, in fact, died shortly after Miriam arrived at home. I am sure she would have been very pleased to have Miriam by her bedside and would have found her a calm and reassuring presence. It turned out that Miriam's mother, Vera, had been diagnosed with cancer nearly a year before but had kept this from her daughter so as not to distract her from her studies—she was very proud that her daughter was going into the profession. I think it was the day after the funeral, or perhaps the second day, that Miriam came back and resumed the course. We had been told about her mother's death and I was shocked to see Miriam back, and as efficient as ever, at work on that day. The word 'resilience' was not in common use then as it is now, but if it had been, Miriam would have made an obvious example of resilience—an exemplar. It seemed that whatever adversity life had in store for her, she, to use the phrase that is often repeated today, bounced back. Others would have succumbed but Miriam appeared to thrive on adversity, like a character in a novel or a play.

Miriam's final year of training, mercifully, went without any further incident.

At the end of the course, a few fellow students decided that nursing was not for them after all and they went on to other careers, one of the very few that I got back in touch with becoming a filmmaker. One failed her exams. Most of us though, some more enthusiastically

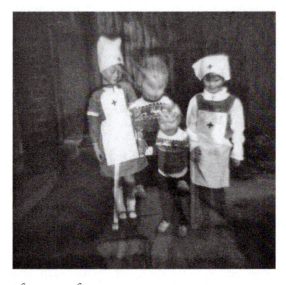

**FIGURE 10.2** Nurse at four years of age

than others, took up offers of jobs on the wards of the hospital that we trained in. The events that I have set down here occurred before nursing courses became university based. Miriam had a reputation for being a star and was offered work on a prestigious ward involved in liver and kidney transplantation under the direction of a pioneering but arrogant transplant surgeon.

The course finished in the summer, which was hot and cloudless, but not as hot as the famous 1976 summer in the UK or the more recent 2018 heat wave. I was able to take two weeks holiday, which I spent mostly lying on a beach on a Greek island reading paperback short stories. I flew back home and, some days before returning to work, found myself walking through the city centre in pleasant sunshine. I noticed, as I was working my way through groups of tourists along St. Andrew's Street, one of the local newspaper stands. Its handwritten headline behind the latticed frame included the word 'nurse'. I think this must have been what drew my attention. I stopped and saw that the headline read 'City Nurse Found Dead'. I remember being only mildly curious and crossed the street to look further. On the top of a pile of folded copies of the [___] *Evening News*, I saw Miriam's name, her full name which I was not used to seeing. This changed the nature of my attention. The story indicated that it was believed that she had died by suicide after returning to her accommodation at the end of a shift by taking an overdose of tablets, which she had apparently been collecting over a period of time. My first thought was that there must be another nurse with the same name as Miriam. In fact, as I carried on toward the market square past the one-man-band busker, I still assumed that this was the case. It was not until the next day and a number of telephone conversations that I discovered—we discovered—that this really concerned the Miriam that we all knew.

At the time, we asked each other how such a confident and calm person could be the same individual who was unhappy enough to take her own life. We rewound the videotapes of our memories of the last years, looking for clues in her behaviour but found nothing.

Today, I say that the story of Miriam has taught me, or rather brought home to me, the fact that the way that someone behaves can tell us very little about how they are responding psychically to events. Some resilience researchers in nursing believe that it is a mark of and is evidence of resilience for a nurse to remain 'at the bedside'. When a nurse leaves the profession, that, they argue, is a sign of a lack of resilience, a kind of failure.

> In our dreams (writes [the poet] Coleridge) images represent the sensations we think they cause; we do not feel horror because we are threatened by a sphinx; we dream of a sphinx in order to explain the horror we feel.
>
> *Borges 2000, p. 276*

# 11

# AN ANONYMOUS STORY

Some time after my first book on resilience was published, I received a piece of writing in the post, anonymously. It arrived in meticulously typewritten script on a bundle of A4 sheets loosely held together with an old-fashioned treasury tag, two hollow little metal tubes kept together by a short piece of red string. At first glance, the documents seemed to me to give an account of a workplace event, or series of events, which the writer saw as enacting an injustice with her as its central victim. A separate note asked that I publicise the story. The bundle contained, along with its narrative content, photocopies of an escalating series of letters of complaint, with the name of the author obscured with liberal layers of thickening Tippex. The first were addressed to a matron in a particular NHS provider. By the end, the anonymous writer had made contact with a Member of Parliament and the Chief Executive of the Nursing and Midwifery Council. Some of the replies were also included. None were sympathetic and none conceded that there was a case to answer. The manuscript arrived at a busy time for me and, after a brief glance, I put it to one side, not sure whether I would take the trouble to retrieve it at a later date. About a year later, when I had started work on this collection, an event occurred, which I will not go into here, that reminded me of the anonymous story and made me both curious about it and uncomfortable that I had not taken the anonymous teller more seriously. I searched it out. This was not straightforward because I had moved office twice since receiving the package and also moved home in the meantime. When eventually I found it, pages were missing, including, unfortunately, the first page or pages. Looking at the text with fresh eyes, I could see that some terrible trauma was described somewhere on those pages. What is left is only a short account of its effect and how the writer responded to it (partly by writing the series of letters of complaint that I mentioned earlier). I wanted to include it in this collection because, even in its fragmented form, it evokes a nurse's struggle to maintain integrity in the face of adversity that seems to span many years.

The tellers of tales of resilience like to present their characters as triumphing over adversity. Who wouldn't? The stories I present in this book, if nothing else, show that it is, in reality, sometimes hard to tell triumph from defeat, and defeat from triumph. Regarding this incomplete tale, I leave it to the reader to decide whether the anonymous writer has 'succumbed' or 'bounced back'.

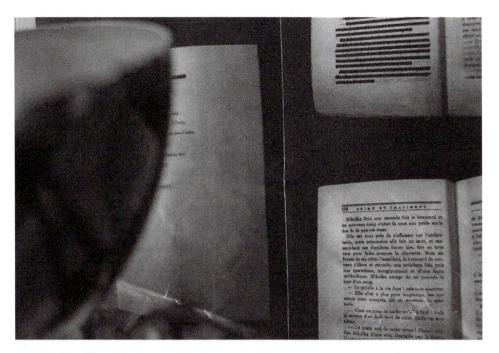

**FIGURE 11.1** Obscured text

'… red stars that I was seeing were the brake lights of the car in front that I realised my eyes were full of tears. I remember thinking at the time, "hold it together". It would really help someone's insurance claim: "the nurse was driving home after a night shift." Also, my reputation would plunge to new lows.

I try to remain strong, but I cry out when I think about it. When I allow myself to get emotional, I could cry non-stop, even now.'

★

'My treatment by the trust over the past three years has damaged my health, my professional reputation and my livelihood. Its effects on my personal and private life have been utterly devastating. You have refused to take my claims seriously throughout.'

★

'I have just read this summary of the dangers of whistle-blowing on a website: "If only whistle-blowing were as simple as taking a deep breath and making a lot of noise. In reality, any nurse who…detects wrongdoing and decides to pursue all avenues necessary to correct it probably is facing a gruelling and complicated task. …the experience can chip away at whistle-blowers' self-worth, and even their faith in humanity. 'It's a very, very dark place for people'…they can lose sleep, have trouble eating or eat too much, struggle socially and become emotionally numb. 'That's why, if you asked them if they were faced with a similar situation, would [they] do things differently, most people say they would just look the other way'" (www.nurse.com/blog/2012/04/02/rn-whistle-blowers-summon-moral-courage/). Yes I know—I was that soldier…'

★

'I remember these strong colours: white and bright red. The white of my uniform under the buzzing fluorescent lights. I walk through a corridor in the middle of the night, between about a quarter to two and five to two, back from the blood bank to the ward. The bags of packed cells are stored in a rotating holder, like a refrigerated version of an old-fashioned Rolodex. I am carrying a bag of crimson blood. How did I get here? Because it is crucial that no one makes a mistake with the administration of blood products, the different types are colour coded, not of much use to those of us who are colour-blind. A nod's as good as a wink. When is it that people die—between three and four in the morning? A nod's as good as a wink to a blind horse.

Just a random statistic to keep you entertained: during the day we had three doctors ready to swoop in to our ward at the first sign of trouble. During the night we share with the whole of the rest of the hospital three of them, all of them as tired as zombies with blood results worse than the patients they treat. Managers, of course, are uncontactable, especially when they know it is me.

The message that *we don't want bad news* infected the whole organisation. There was absolutely no moral compass. The managers all wore horrible clothes.'

★

'The counsels at the NMC, young women, all wear black skirts and jackets, white blouses, tan tights and low-heeled—no other word but sensible—black shoes. Certainly not crimson high-heeled shoes. They don't even have a pair under the bed at home to wear on a night out. When did I last have a night out? They call one another "my learned friend". A melancholy legal bod sits to the right of the chair, wincing with irritation every now and then. There is a labelled desk for the witness and, directly opposite them, a shorthand writer fills a growing pile of spiral notebooks with what appears to be real shorthand. Yours truly, of course, is there, sitting like Nelly between a union representative, who leaves at lunchtime, thank you for nothing, and counsel. Oh, I forgot to say, this is three years later.

He worked on the railway all his life, they said.

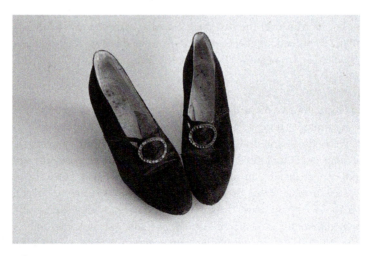

**FIGURE 11.2** Shoes

Lunchtime. I'll spare you the details of the morning, the long discussions about the evidence and the quiet sniggering of a line of my ex-colleagues in the public seats exchanging grins. The public seats at the coliseum. Christians and slaves battle with the lions. Lunchtime. But then the defendant's counsel calls Nelly to the witness bench and I am not too stupid to notice that everything changes. Those in the room learn first that, during the time running up to "the incident" on nightshift, Nelly here was being beaten by her vicious partner as their relationship irretrievably broke down. And not sleeping during the days because of this. The counsel asks for further detail of the events leading up to the incident. Then they are really shocked and so they should be: in the previous year, yours truly had a brain tumour removed from the folds of her delicate white matter and then picked up a nasty dose of meningitis after the surgery, just when I thought I was getting over it. At work, I had been "phased back" like the phases of the moon, waning, gibbous, lost behind clouds, over the preceding months. I had agreed to the plan they offered me.'

★

'I try to remain strong, but I cry out when I think about it. When I allow myself to get emotional I could cry non-stop, even now.'

★

'Dear managers,
    You were keen to be seen to be acting properly. Nobody can fault you for that. You upheld the reputation of the Trust and you have an admirable sense of unity among yourselves.
    Yours sincerely.'

★

'I didn't need a stick any more but my colleagues helpfully told me that, when I was upset or I cried, which I did a lot, surprise, surprise, that I sounded a bit like a pig. Sometimes it was another farmyard animal. Nobody wanted to work a shift with me. I could perfectly well see my colleagues roll their eyes when they were allocated to work an end with me. The solution I found—night duty. Another way to safety: I decided to adopt an attitude of meek semi-acquiescence. But I knew there was a disaster waiting to happen and I made sure the right people knew it too. '

★

'Dear [___], M.P.,
    I am writing to ask whether you are aware of the dangerous shortage of nursing staff at ___ _ Hospital in your constituency. This shortage has been drawn to the attention of managers at all levels and to the Chief Executive of [___], all without satisfactory response.
    Yours sincerely.
    PS. My next letter is to the [___], our local newspaper, which is not averse to featuring stories about [___] Hospital on its front page.'

★

'Phased return to work. Sorry to return to this but can someone please explain to me how phased works with probably three down on every shift? And, can you just cover this? You don't mind, do you?'

★

The final page of the whole document takes the form of a copy of a letter addressed to the Chief Executive and Registrar of the NMC. I do not know if it was ever sent and, if it was, whether it was responded to:

'Dear NMC,

Thank you for dealing with my situation on [date] and for finding that I had no case to answer. Thank you for saying that it was regrettable that it had taken over three years for my hearing to happen. Thank you for telling the court that my return to work should have been managed better and that I should have been offered more support by my employer. Thank you for telling me that I was free to work as a nurse, subject to completing an approved Return to Practice programme.

I would like to inform you that I have not worked as a nurse since I was suspended nearly four years ago and that I have no plan to work as a nurse again.

Yours sincerely.'

Then, added as a PS: 'Finally, can I suggest that you take my precious PIN [a nurse's personal registration number] and place it somewhere about your person where the sun don't shine.'

Despite the anonymous writer's regrettable lack of respect for the profession's regulator, reading through and attempting to make sense of her dossier led me toward a relatively unsystematic perusal of the records not only of NMC hearings but of those of the Medical Practitioner Tribunal Service, which sits in judgement over whether individual doctors are fit to practise. The records of the charges against nurses and doctors seem to largely fall into two groups. The first concerns matters of dishonesty, sometimes involving financial gain for those involved. The second concerns practice failures. Of those concerning practice failures, some appear, from a reading of the evidence presented, to feature mention of adverse circumstances for the individual involved. This might take the form of working already extended shifts that then overrun, unexpected absences of colleagues, IT failures, conflicting clinical priorities or working in organisations under investigation. The NMC tells us 'In cases where a nurse or midwife's fitness to practise is alleged to be impaired by reason of health then the hearing will be held in private due to the confidential nature of these cases.' (www.nmc.org.uk/concerns-nurses-midwives/hearings/our-panels-case-examiners/fitness-to-practise-committee/)   In the case described here, the health of the anonymous teller was clearly an important aspect of the story, although it is also apparent that the case was not held in private. I did not come upon any cases where interpersonal difficulties or the unpopularity of the registrant with colleagues or with managers were considered as contributing factors, at least in the written records. Clearly, these factors play a part in the story presented here and possibly in other cases. I did not look at every case, of course.

It is also claimed that whistle-blowers can end up themselves being disciplined or even struck off (Empey 2004, Fagan 2004). One prominent example concerns the nurse who secretly filmed instances of patient neglect in a hospital ward in the south of England for the BBC television documentary series Panorama (BBC One Web Team Blog 2009). The NMC accused her of breaching patient confidentiality by working secretly for Panorama and she was struck off the register. Following an outpouring of support from the public and a petition of over 40,000 signatures calling for her reinstatement, her sentence was reduced to a one-year caution and she was able to return to practice.

The nameless nurse at the heart of this chapter made the decision not to return.

# 12

# YASMIN, THE NURSE WHO WAS BULLIED AND WHO BIT BACK

This is a story about nurses and bullying. It is not an easy story to hear. I included some pages about this topic in my last book on resilience.[1] I wrote about how bullying can turn a confident and good-humoured professional or a highly motivated student into a self-doubting mess, unable to sleep or make decisions. I also set out the action, both formal and personal, that someone who is experiencing bullying can take. What I didn't write was that the account on those pages was given life by conversations I had had with one particular ward sister I am calling, in this chapter, Yasmin. If you are toward the lower end of nursing's professional hierarchy, you may think of those in these clinical management jobs as comfortable, confident, powerful even. But if you are in these roles yourself, or have been, you know that their level of responsibility brings a new visibility and an entirely new vulnerability. Wherever you are in a hierarchy, there is someone who can make your working life miserable. What Yasmin told me during two meetings in a café close, but not too close, to the hospital where she worked, and later more formally, became the basis for the comments about bullying and what to do about it in that earlier book. Here, I have returned to Yasmin's first-person account of her difficult experiences and her own words to present this uncomfortable story. But first, a summary of what we know about bullying at work.

When organisations like an NHS trust have to operate with reducing budgets or with threats of budget cuts, there is bound to be an impact. Managers who, on a good day, are humane and conscientious may end up making unpalatable decisions in the almost impossible position of having to maintain services with inadequate budgets. Detecting inefficiency and waste can only go so far. Senior managers restructure their organisations to try to wipe off costs. In reorganisations, it is often middle-level managers who are made redundant or moved to other less attractive posts. In NHS trusts, wards or units can be merged to save the salary of a ward manager or two. There is nearly always an effect on people's lives. The sudden loss of both your income and position, as well as anxiety about this being about to happen, can alter people's behaviour, sometimes dramatically. Cultures of uncertainty, anxiety and resentment

---

1 Chapter 7: Being a student, being a worker. See from page 110 onwards. Some of that content is summarised here.

can develop. One report from Cranfield School of Management into the well-known scandal at Stafford hospital in the 2000s comments in particular on the predicament of middle managers, like unit-level managers, in 'low-trust, low-autonomy' environments (Buchanan, Denyer et al. 2013). When middle managers are placed under pressure or feel they have no control over decision-making that involves their own staff, these pressures can seep into the most vulnerable places in their psyche. Those who are prone to a sense of powerlessness can become resentful and embittered. Others can turn to harsh and dictatorial approaches as a way of coping with their own insecurities about their status and position. In a review of bullying at work, the British Psychological Society tells us that the majority of bullying is done by managers and that younger workers, who may be unaware of their workplace rights, as well as members of ethnic minorities—like Yasmin—are the most vulnerable to bullying (Cartwright and Cooper 2007). Yasmin, it is clear, was at the receiving end of such a culture and of such behaviour.

We met, on a windy day, in a coffee chain store. This particular branch had more than its fair share of deep leather sofas and armchairs. The screams of an insistent alarm on some piece of catering equipment bit into our conversation every three to four minutes. In the end, we stopped noticing this intrusion as we sat opposite each other at one end of a long table and Yasmin's story deepened. A grandmother with a baby was handing it over to its newly arrived mother who bounced it up and down on a small table near us and mouthed to it expressively while it gnawed on a finger with its as yet toothless gums. I remember starting to notice my own toothache from a filling done the week before. A bus outside stopped on the hill was parked at such a sloping angle that it had a disconcerting effect on us, as if the world outside were gradually sliding downwards and beyond our reach. There was something fragile about many of the coffee-drinking clients around us. An elderly man with white hair and a wispy white beard, who arrived wearing very dark sunglasses that he did not take off, and his companion in a baseball cap dropped their lunches and coffees on the floor while attempting to change tables, leaving a puddle of froth on the ground, which they tried to scoop up with napkins. A father with a teenage son using a stick for walking, both of them in black anoraks, came in and went out while we were talking. Someone was enviably asleep in an alcove, deep in a heavy coat, the fake fur collar up around the top of their head. Yasmin's story starts with her making a mistake, a relatively small mistake.

'I was asked to do an audit of staff and non-staff costs in the ward over the past year. It was complicated and the information was hard to get hold of. I had to rely on two or three financial people to help me and I was late in sending it to the manager for our site. After I had submitted it to him, I realised that I had put down some of the expenses to the wrong cost centre. So I redid three of the tables and sent those in to him, asking him to disregard the last report I'd sent. But for some reason, they either did not get my revised work, or got it too late, and I was called in to see him. The Head of Finance was also at the meeting, which surprised me because I thought it was just a routine meeting. They told me that I had attempted to hide some of my expenditure on the ward. They said that they had looked back at my accounting over the last three years and told me that I had been hiding costs repeatedly. They told me that I had committed fraud and that they would be starting a formal disciplinary process and that I could be dismissed. The case might even be reported to the police. I was confused and flustered. I had always been conscientious and worked to the very best of my ability. I was always staying late to make sure everything was organised. My staff always spoke highly of me. No one had ever cast doubt on my abilities or my honesty before. This came as an utter shock. When I had

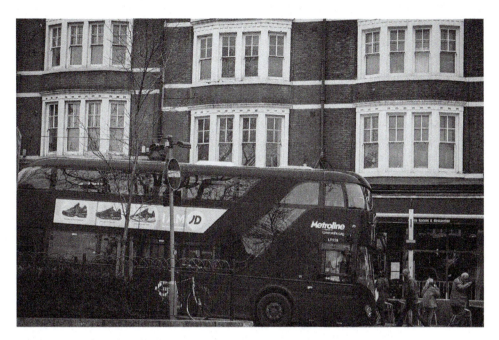

**FIGURE 12.1** Tilting bus

regained some composure, I went back through every record I could find of how I'd managed my budget. There were three or four errors, it's true, but they were all for small amounts like £40 or £62 and were the kind of items you could either code as supplies or equipment and I had been inconsistent. I copied all the accounts and pointed out my mistakes and I sent them to John [the unit manager] with an explanation. I received no response. I forwarded them to the Head of Finance and also received no reply. A week went by and neither of them replied. I left phone messages for John to try to arrange to see him to explain but he never got back to me. I couldn't help feeling that they were playing with me and that their silence was part of the game. I never did receive any formal notice of a disciplinary nor any other formal communication but, in less than two weeks, dwelling on this, I was already planning to resign. I would never have believed that this single event could have such an effect on me.'

'They say that being bullied increases the risk of abusing alcohol and drugs. It's true. After evenings of drinking wine, I would find myself running my fingernails over a blister pack of Zopiclone that I found in my bathroom cupboard—I don't remember how it got there—just to make sure I didn't wake up in the night still thinking about it. In those evenings, I would look around my rooms, at the dishes in the kitchen, at the trinkets in my bedroom that used to give me small warm feelings as my eye rolled over them, at a packet of cotton buds, at the television turned off. All of these things, everything I looked at, was lit by a new harsh light, like the police shining a torch around my flat after a murder or searching for a criminal. Nothing in these homely things gave me any comfort. That horrible experience at work had reached right into my home and bleached away its homeliness.'

'I have gone over and over in my head what they said to me and what I should have said back to them. I can't stop reliving this'.

I asked Yasmin how the story had played out.

'A family friend is an employment lawyer, so I spoke to her about this. She told me that it was completely ridiculous and unfounded to describe my errors as fraud and that they should have made clear, in advance, the nature of the meeting that they called me to. It clearly was not a formal disciplinary meeting. So that helped a little, but it did not make me less angry. And I never had any apology. It affected my work. I realised I was snappy in a way I had never been before. But I slowly began to realise that there was a pattern of behaviour toward me. I realised that I was always asked to justify any requests to go on training courses, while others never seemed to have to. I realised that other less experienced and less qualified sisters had been promoted and that my applications never got further than interviews. I think, basically, that being Asian, my face just did not fit in with all the senior managers who were white and most were men. I know I should have some distance now from what happened but, I have to be honest, it is slow to get over my hate and fear for those two and until recently I've still felt a sense of vulnerability when I think about it. I've moved now, to another unit, and that's better, but I know I will leave eventually. I'm hopeful that I can put this behind me and flourish. I know I can now.'

I asked Yasmin what had happened, what had helped her to develop this 'resilience'?

The bus rolled off down the hill. The mother and the baby left. One of the waitresses brought out a folding yellow hazard sign and started mopping the spilled food and drinks from the floor. Yasmin was silent for a long time and then replied.

'Well, strangely, on one of the nights when I couldn't sleep, I turned on the television. I hope you don't mind me telling you this. I usually watched Fear Files on ZEE TV, but there was a film showing, it turned out to be quite a gruesome horror film—it was very late—and I never watch horror films. It was about a teenage woman and the men she encountered. She had a particular, er, condition. It was stupid but I fell asleep watching it. I dreamed I was that girl. In the dream, I was on a bed in a room. It was someone's flat, and it was a complete mess, and there was a fierce dog barking in a cage close by. I was having sex with someone. It was the finance director, only he had tattoos down his back. At some point, while we were making love, I remembered that my vagina had teeth, strong sharp teeth. The camera zoomed in on me smiling to myself. Then, I used my teeth. All those pelvic floor exercises stood me in good stead. I bit twice, hard, and screechy violins started playing. He stared into my eyes for some time, then he started violently shaking and pulled away shocked and bewildered. He started looking around the room as if for something he had lost. The dog had stopped barking and

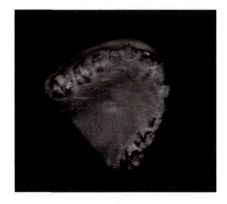

**FIGURE 12.2** Teeth

was now whining loudly. I climbed off the bed and, as I stood up, the lost object slid onto the floor with an unforgettable sound. Then I woke up. I woke up strangely calm after such a weird dream. Strangely, strangely confident. I started, just started, to have the feeling that whatever the adversity, I could be a match to it. It was a new dawn. Ah, I've just remembered—that was the name of the girl in the film.'

At the end of our meeting, we shook hands and Yasmin walked boldly out of the café leaving me to write up my notes. I do not think that Yasmin had ever told her dream to anyone and, to be honest, I found myself unsettled by its content. The waitress folded up the yellow hazard sign and wheeled the bucket and mop back into the storeroom. I decided against another coffee. I was thinking, for some reason, about those lists of sources of resilience that I had read so many times.

# 13

# MARTA, THE MIGRANT NURSE

Marta was a migrant nurse. She never once told me, while she was alive, about the prejudice and suspicion that she must have faced on her arrival in this country. In a sense, though, it was plain to see.

Migration and nursing have gone hand in hand since the profession's early days. At an individual level, a nursing qualification has been seen as a ticket to travel, to take, perhaps, an extended gap year before settling down to more long term employment at home. On the system level, however, international nurse migration is more troublesome. At this level, it is clear that migration can be motivated by the desire for a better standard of living, better career and educational opportunities and even the need for personal safety. But it has harmful effects because rich nations like the UK and United States look to recruit from less developed countries with already low levels of nurses per population to meet their own nurse shortages. The UK in particular suffers from a cyclical shortage of nurses, a result of policy decisions influencing the number of budgeted nurse posts, as well as fluctuations in investment in nurse education reflecting overall economic variation (Pittman, Aiken et al. 2007). The early 2000s, and more recently the mid 2010s have both witnessed recruitment drives to plug shortages or facilitate expansions in nursing numbers in the UK health service.

But nurses from overseas, like any migrants, can face difficulties. This can take the form of racism, prejudice and xenophobia that are present in general society, alongside specific professional barriers, sometimes to registration in the UK (Allan, Cowie et al. 2009). Like the nurses recruited from the West Indies in the 1940s and 1950s, and those more recently recruited from within the European Union, they are both welcomed and unwelcome. That racist attacks, verbal and physical, on EU migrants increased following the UK referendum vote to leave the EU is evidence that some people do not like foreigners and that sometimes the talk of politicians can embolden racists (Dearden 2017). The election of Donald Trump in the US in 2017 and the vote to leave the European Union in the UK in 2016 suggest that, in these two countries at least, migrants might not be quite as welcome as they were, despite both countries' historic reliance on both skilled and unskilled migrant workers.

The NHS and, more recently, universities have set up initiatives to support overseas recruited nurses, both in their employment and in their personal lives in this country. Employers and those involved in nurse education now realise that all does not necessarily go smoothly for nurse migrants.

So Marta's story is a story shared by countless nurses over the years and over the globe. The time immediately following the Second World War (1939–45) marked a period of ambitious economic expansion in the UK as the nation sought to re-establish its peacetime economy. In addition, the National Health Service, founded in 1948, needed a supply of workers to staff it. The stories of recruitment and migration from the West Indies, initially via the *Empire Windrush* that arrived in Tilbury docks in London in June 1948 (see Chapter 8), are well known along with the discrimination that many black migrants faced. Not so well known is the story of recruitment in the late 1940s and 1950s from Germany (and Sudetenland, parts of the present Czech and Slovak republics), very recently the UK's wartime enemy. The experiences of this group of migrants are told in few places (Weber-Newth and Steinert 2006).[1] The 'North Sea Scheme', among many others, was particularly aimed at bringing young German women to the UK. In addition to the economic drivers, the government also sought to make the humanitarian and magnanimous gestures of the victor of the war. The scheme started in summer 1948. In July of that year, the Ministry of Labour issued a press release stating that a number of German women would be coming to the UK as domestic staff for hospitals and other sectors. By the end of August, 4,000 women had already applied and been accepted. The women had to be between 18 and 28 years old. They were not permitted to bring family members. The first group of 50 German student nurses arrived in Britain on 15th August 1948. By 1950, a little over 9,500 had arrived in Britain. Among them were approximately 775 student nurses and 59 trained nurses.

Both 'push' and 'pull' factors were involved in migration from Germany to the UK. But, like many migrants, Marta had her own personal reasons for leaving home. She was born and grew up in the Ruhr, the industrial and coal-mining region of Germany, in the northwest of the country. Although the town that she lived in was known as 'Die Goldene Stadt' (The Golden City) because of the comparatively limited damage suffered from bombing during World War II, her mother had died in 1942, she told me, of a brain haemorrhage following the sound of a large explosion nearby. Marta was 18 and received a phone call while at work.

'They called the doctor and the doctor said, "get an ambulance". She was taken to the hospital but she was dead. I went to work because we had to start before seven. I just got there and I had to go back. My mother was 43. My sister was 14.'

Her father, a coalmine worker, later remarried. Marta did not get on with her stepmother it seems—in some photographs that she showed me while we talked, she certainly appeared unsmiling and stern. Perhaps Marta already had a sense that she would leave the country. She told me that, while working as a secretary, she learned English and with one week's pay bought a suitcase and had photos taken for a passport. As her name suggests, she had some Polish relatives who had moved to the Ruhr a generation or two earlier.

When the North Sea Scheme was announced, she was ready to go. She started her journey at an assembly centre specifically for young women on this scheme near Münster, 50 kilometres from where she lived. She stayed there for three days. Applicants were examined by a doctor and their luggage was checked by customs. The women were given £1 pocket money for the voyage. On the third day, they were put onto a train from Marienthal, Münster, to the Hook of Holland to board the overnight boat to Harwich, on the Essex coast. Their journey mirrored

---

1 Unless otherwise stated, statistics in this chapter come from this source.

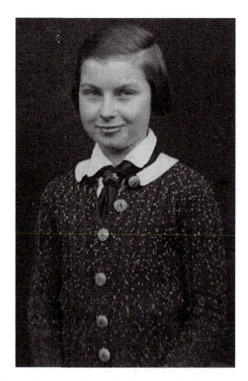

**FIGURE 13.1** Young migrant nurse

those that other less fortunate individuals had been forced to take during the previous years. Marta remembers the smuts from the ship's funnels falling on her white coat as she boarded the boat at night, the bunk beds of her cabin and being sick on the journey. This was the same route used by the Kindertransport ten years earlier, a rescue effort that took place during the months prior to the outbreak of the Second World War. The UK took in nearly 10,000 predominantly Jewish unaccompanied children from Germany, Austria, Czechoslovakia and Poland (https://en.wikipedia.org/wiki/Kindertransport).[2]

Generally, the women did not know in advance what kind of work they would be doing once they arrived. Marta and her friend Gerda were sent to Bracebridge Heath mental hospital near Lincoln. It was renamed St. Johns Hospital in the 1960s before being closed in the late 1980s or early 1990s and left empty until a housing development took place on the site. Its grand Italian-style shell attracted urban explorers who gain access to and photograph derelict institutions.[3] In the early days of the NHS, jobs there were difficult to fill with local labour and the practice of recruiting foreigners, who might be less choosy because of their own extreme circumstances, was adopted by the health service as a short-term solution to recruitment. The fact that many

2 *Austerlitz*, by the German novelist W. G. Sebald, is the story of a Kindertransport boy brought up in an inhospitable Welsh manse who later traces his origins to Prague and then goes back there, retracing his journey by train, travelling via Austerlitz station in Paris.
3 See   www.bcd-urbex.com/st-johns-hospital-aka-county-pauper-lunatic-asylum-lincoln/.   Forgotten   and abandoned places often hold stunning architecture, left to decay. The art of visiting forgotten places is called Urban Exploring, or Urbex for short.

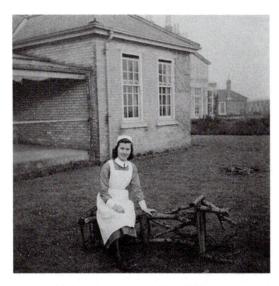

**FIGURE 13.2** Migrant nurse

migrants of the same nationality were employed in the same institution created possibilities for camaraderie. Marta received a distant friendliness from English colleagues. In our discussion, she was reluctant to talk about suspicion and overt racism, but I think these can be read between the lines of what she told me. Accounts from other migrants make it clear that both occurred.

'It was good to get my own room. I did not have this even at home. There were fireplaces, stoves and hot water. But there was not enough fresh air. The windows were open just a little bit at the top. And we had decent uniforms.'

After a short training period, Marta learned on the job.

'I did not know anything about what a nurse had to do. The nurses who had worked there for a long time showed us what to do. We had to clean the ward, help wash the patients, take temperatures and serve meals. I learned to do bandaging and to test how hot the water in a bath was by dipping my elbow in. We went to training school for three months, where we learned practical things like how to make beds. After a few more months, we were allowed to give out medicine and write in the patients' notes. Making beds was difficult with all those blankets. We did not have blankets at home. We had an eiderdown. We thought England was old-fashioned.'

'What did the patients think of having a German nurse?'

'They liked us. Some were so grateful, they would give us chocolate or cigarettes. That wasn't allowed but they did it all the same. It was the patients who made you know you were doing a good job.'

'Did you smoke then?'

'Everybody smoked then.'

'And what about the nurses in charge?'

'There was discipline. It was very strict. Some of them, you heard, did not like Germans but I was fine. They were nice to me because I was in a special group'.[4]

4 Marta was part of the 'Scheme for Training German Girls as State Registered Nurses in Great Britain' (Public Records Office 1949).

There was a huge demand for nurses. In the late 1940s, approximately 22,000 individuals started training each year but less than half completed their course. German students had additional requirements over and above indigenous recruits. They had to be between 18 and 25 years old, have a 'good education' and have a high standard of written and spoken English. They had to commit themselves to complete the course (Public Records Office 1949). Despite this, there were great pressures.

'We were put onto night shift very soon. So we worked five nights and then two nights off but instead of going to bed, which you wanted to do, we had to go to lessons in the classroom.'

'How did you spend your time off?'

'Mostly we met in each other's rooms—even though that wasn't allowed. We cheered up anyone who was homesick or who was saying that they wanted to leave. Coming up to Christmas, we sung carols in German. That cheered us up too.'

Nursing work also gave Marta a sense of status and her wages gave her independence and self-reliance during her time here before her marriage.

Marta did not want to talk about how or when she met her husband. All she said was that he was a British soldier still serving and stationed in Lincoln at the time. When I asked whether they had met at a tea dance, popular during and after the Second World War, she gave an evasive answer. I was hoping to hear some fond memories of that period in her life. I believe that she married in 1950 and I know that her husband died in 1996, aged 76, after a second heart attack brought on by an accident on a train. She had two children. Marta was also unwilling to talk about any prejudice or discrimination that she might have faced on her arrival in England or at any time thereafter. Her acute discomfort at my questions suggested to me that it was still an issue that affected her deeply. I knew from my reading about the period that discrimination against Germans was common. Some Germans were refused service in pubs, some had swastikas painted on their front doors and some had death threats made over the telephone. A little later, the children of some German migrants were teased at school or forced to play the role of a Nazi in playground games. During the 1960s, children's comics regularly featured cruel Germans in military uniforms and recognisable Nazi helmets repeating words like 'Schweinehund', 'Achtung' and 'Gott in Himmel!'. This widely circulating media cannot have made it easy for the children of German migrants. When I asked whether Marta spoke German at home to her children when they were small, her brief answer was 'no'.

'What about German cooking?'

'I used to buy Frankfurter sausages sometimes'.

It seemed very clear that Marta, like some other German migrants, felt acutely conspicuous of being 'the enemy' and did all she could to avoid notice. The period between their arrival in the late 1940s and the end of the 1960s was widely seen as the most difficult for German migrants. After this period, with the perhaps more tolerant society of the 1970s, many were able to settle into new lives, most with British husbands. Marta left nursing at this time and started work for a pharmaceutical company in Greenford in Middlesex. She worked there until her retirement. She told me that she returned to Germany for her father's funeral but she kept in touch with very few family members and fewer German friends.

But what has Marta to say about her years growing up in Nazi Germany, the elephant in the room of our conversation? She tells me two contradictory stories. In the first, she is a young girl and sees a Hitler doll in a shop window but her parents disapprove and refuse to buy it for her. In the second, she tells me that, of course, at a young age, she was a member of the Hitler Youth.

'I don't know what all the fuss is about. All we did was embroidery.'

And what about immediately after the end of the war, in the devastation of a ruined and defeated country? She tells me another two incidents, without emotion. It was the Americans who moved into and occupied her part of Germany. A local man in the home guard remained loyal to the Nazis. His neighbours told him to throw away his rifle but he refused and was shot by the allies. Marta remembers that he was a schoolteacher. She remembers looking at the American GIs and that this was the first time in her life that she had seen a black person.

Marta was in her late seventies when I talked to her about this time in her life and her experience of nursing. She died a week after her eightieth birthday, of mesothelioma. Is her story one of resilience? If it is, it had a personal cost for her. Circumstances conspired to separate her from her family and her German identity and to teach her above all to avoid notice. But she worked hard to establish herself and her family and contributed her wages to buy a large detached suburban house, though in the end I sensed that her material advances counted for very little in the face of what she had given up. She never appeared to reflect on or at least talk openly about her early life, growing up during wartime, or her experience of migration and I wonder if this inability eventually led to a kind of despair and bitterness.

I close this chapter and this part of the book with the eulogy that I read at her funeral:

> Mum was born in Germany in May 1925. She was the daughter of a miner. She grew up in one of the most turbulent times in Europe and in one of the most bombed parts of Germany. Shortly after the Second World War ended, she learned English and spent her first salary on a suitcase. She made the decision to immigrate to England where prospects would have been rather brighter. On arrival she lived in Lincoln where she trained to be a nurse. She met my father there shortly afterwards and the two got married in 1950. He was in the army at that time. They moved to London a year or so later and lived in barracks until they bought their first house in Greenford, and their second here in Ruislip in 1970. My mother's legacy is hard work. She worked continuously until she retired in 1985 and, partly as a result, she enabled her family to grow up with comforts and opportunities that neither her, nor my father's parents, would have dreamed of. She leaves two children and three grandchildren.

# PART III

# 14

# HOW TO USE THE STORIES

In this final chapter, I have gathered together pointers to background material that is relevant to each chapter, along with a series of questions and topics for discussion in the classroom or for personal reflection.

## Carole, the nurse who went on strike

According to UNISON, the UK's largest union, 'Trade unions are groups of employees who join together to maintain and improve their conditions of employment' (www.unison.org.uk/about/what-we-do/about-trade-unions/). Workplaces in various sectors often recognise particular unions that they work with, for example to discuss major redundancies or health and safety issues, and to negotiate pay, of course. The RCN, likely to be most familiar to nurses and healthcare assistants in the UK, describes itself as both a professional body and a trade union. It became a trade union in 1976. The RCN has some particular features: it has a Royal Charter[1] and is a member, along with fourteen other unions, of the NHS Staff Council, which negotiates pay and terms and conditions for NHS staff. Although you might expect a professional body and the professional regulator—for nurses and midwives, this is the NMC—to work closely together and have similar objectives, in some ways they have, and have to be seen to have, opposing missions. The professional body works in the interests of the profession and its members. They pay its bills after all. The regulator works to safeguard the public and prominent among its roles is that of policing the profession's members. Actually, those same members also pay the bills of the NMC.

## Questions

- Are you a member of a trade union? If so, why? And if not, why not?
- Do you know your union's policy about strike action and about action short of a strike?

---

1 The Royal Charter was granted in 1929. Before that, it had the more prosaic name of College of Nursing Limited.

- In May 2017, the RCN balloted members about whether they would strike in support of the union's pay claim. Four out of five voted for strike action, but do you know what proportion of the RCN membership voted?
- Would you ever consider striking?
- What action short of a strike would be possible for you in your own work setting?
- Do you know what the NMC's position on industrial action is?

## Reading

Find out about the history of trades unions at Wikipedia: https://en.wikipedia.org/wiki/Trade_union
Charlesworth, A. and S. Lafond (2017). "Shifting from undersupply to oversupply: Does NHS workforce planning need a paradigm shift?" *Economic Affairs* **37**(1): 36–52.
Traynor, M. (2013). *Nursing in Context: policy politics profession*. Basingstoke, Palgrave.

## Beverley, the student nurse who refused to fear

This story has styles of pedagogy and their effects at its heart. Beverley tells how a particular pedagogy that she encountered had the effect of being profoundly disempowering—inadvertently. Her story seems to show that although she found the experience initially isolating, after a little inquiry she found that others in her class shared her feeling.

### Questions

- If you are a student nurse, can you think of examples of elements of your course that imply a cultural norm, how a nurse is expected to behave or dress for example?
- Do you think fundamental beliefs about professional life emerge from any particular set of cultural values? Or are they value-neutral?
- Do you think anything about the way your university course, or workplace, is organised makes things more difficult for you because of your particular ethnic or cultural identity?
- Does the ethnic mix of tutors (if you are a student) reflect that of your fellow students?
- Does the ethnic mix of managers (if you are a qualified nurse or a nurse lecturer yourself) in your area reflect that of your fellow nurses or colleagues?

## Reading

For an analysis of the key differences between the two similar-sounding terms 'critical thinking' and 'critical pedagogy', see:
Burbules, N. and R. Berk (1999). "Critical Thinking and Critical Pedagogy: Relations, Differences, and Limits." In *Critical theories in education*. T. Popkewitz and L. Fendler (Eds.). New York, Routledge.
For a recent general text on critical pedagogy, see:
Dyson, S. (2018). *Critical Pedagogy in Nursing*. Basingstoke, Palgrave Macmillan.

## Laura, student nurses and 'real' nurses

This story looks at an aspect of professional socialisation through the eyes of a small group of student nurses, and particularly one now-qualified nurse who looks back on her thoughts before she qualified. I think it is fair to say that nurse training, as an instance of professional socialisation, will have episodes of difficulty, and Laura talks about the effects of this difficulty on her personal life. She is, however, positive about the experience and has realistic ideas of how change might be introduced. Her story suggests that having a broad understanding of how health service issues affect personal behaviour can, if not insulate the individual from distress, go a long way to making that distress less overwhelming. The extracts from the focus group show how different individuals can have very different responses to similar experiences.

## Questions

- What is meant by the term professional socialisation?
- The focus group shows that, while most of the students appear to agree with each other's views about qualified nurses' behaviour, one or two do not. How would you account for such wide differences in response?
- If you are a nurse, can you think of instances when you were acting as a mentor but were thwarted in the role by lack of time and feeling under pressure? Assuming you answered 'yes' (!), how did you deal with that situation?
- If you are a student nurse who feels that a mentor has not given you the attention that you required, how was that dealt with between you? If this has happened more than once, how did different mentors approach this?

## Reading

Allan, H., M. Traynor, D. Kelly and P. Smith (2016). "Becoming a Nurse." *Understanding Sociology in Nursing*. London, Sage: 50–70.

O'Driscoll, M. F., H. T. Allan and P. A. Smith (2010). "Still looking for leadership—Who is responsible for student nurses' learning in practice?" *Nurse education today* **30**(3): 212–217.

Maben, J., S. Latter and J. M. Clark (2007). "The sustainability of ideals, values and the nursing mandate: evidence from a longitudinal qualitative study." *Nursing Inquiry* **14**(2): 99–113.

## Polly, the student nurse who wrote poetry and went missing

We might ask ourselves: What is a nurse? What is poetry?

I think we can safely assume that we all know more or less what a nurse is, but what about poetry? What defines a poem, apart from the fact that the lines often don't make it to the end of the page? Modernist[2] poet T. S. Eliot wrote, in his essay on Tradition and the Individual Talent:

> Poetry is not a turning loose of emotion, but an escape from emotion; it is not the expression of personality, but an escape from personality. But, of course, only those who have personality and emotions know what it means to want to escape from these things.
>
> *Eliot 1919*

2 Wikipedia tells us: "For the modernist [poets], it was essential to move away from the merely personal towards an intellectual statement that poetry could make about the world. Even when they reverted to the personal, like T. S. Eliot in the *Four Quartets* and Ezra Pound in *The Cantos*, they distilled the personal into a poetic texture that claimed universal human significance (https://en.wikipedia.org/wiki/Modernist_poetry). I mention this because it gives some explanation for Eliot's statement.

Despite Eliot's note of cultural snobbery, what is worth discussing about this statement on poetry is his refusal to paint a picture of poetry as a kind of spontaneous and individualistic outpouring of emotion. For him, and others, the best poetry is as intellectually rigorous as it is emotionally intense.

## Questions

- Thinking about Polly, the subject of this chapter, how far was her turn to poetry an escape from emotion or an expression of emotion?
- Looking at the three poems of hers that are included in this chapter, would you say that this changes over the course of time?
- Do you think that her poetry gets better?

## Reading

You can find a great many resources about the intersection of nursing work and poetry and general storytelling. An accessible starting point is this recording of an International Nurses Day talk by Charley Barker: www.youtube.com/watch?v=Q9uJG5Wd4cY.

Madeleine Mysco, a graduate of The Writing Seminar series at The Johns Hopkins University in the United States, gives a first-person account of being a nurse: www.rattle.com/when-the-poet-happens-to-be-a-nurse-by-madeleine-mysko/.

The following publications address the same topic with varying degrees of insight and usefulness:

Davis, C. (1997) "Poetry about patients: Hearing the nurse's voice." *Journal of Medical Humanities* 18(2), 111–125.

Jack, K. (2015) "The use of poetry writing in nurse education: An evaluation." *Nurse Education Today* 35(9), e7–e10.

Speare, J. and Henshall, A. (2014) "'Did anyone think the trees were students?' Using poetry as a tool for critical reflection." *Reflective Practice: International and Multidisciplinary Perspectives.* 15(6), 1–14.

## Simone, the nurse who stood in solidarity: working on the border between religion, madness and profession

The long title of this story gives an indication of the range of topics that it includes. The main topic is the requirement of professionals like nurses to work with clients who have particular religious beliefs and practices that the nurse does not share. The converse challenge is for the practitioner to work in a way that does not submit their clients and patients to unwanted expressions of their own religious beliefs and practices. Records of the NMC's fitness to practice hearings, where decisions are made about whether to impose various disciplines on registrants, include cases of such unwanted expressions. Alongside this topic in this chapter is a less concrete but nevertheless pressing concern about what motivates nurses in their work. For many nurses it is the deep-seated belief that they are 'making a difference' to patients and clients. But what if the rug is pulled out from under this cherished belief and the nurse is forced to re-evaluate the impact that their practice is having on clients? This is the challenge that Simone rises to in this story. Her response is what makes it a story about resilience. Like a broken umbrella in the wind and rain, it can sometimes come as a great relief to discard something that you thought, once, would give you shelter.

## Questions

- In your practice, have you come across patients or clients whose expression of their religious faith has made working with them complex? How did you and your team respond?
- Do you think Simone could have done anything that would have avoided her practising/behaving in a way that some of her clients did not appreciate?
- In your work life, have you ever had a sudden realisation that things are not how you thought they were? Can you remember in detail what this experience felt like and what you did about it?
- What is your main motivation to nurse? Would you still nurse without this central motivation? And if you would, how would things be different?

## Reading

Department of Health (2009) *Religion or Belief: a Practical Guide for the NHS*. Available at: www. clatterbridgecc.nhs.uk/application/files/7214/3445/0178/ReligionorbeliefApracticalguideforthe NHS.pdf. Though not new, this booklet gives basic advice about how religion and beliefs affect recruitment, training and work practices in the NHS, as well as implications for treating patients.

Reinert, K. G. and H. G. Koenig (2013). "Re-examining definitions of spirituality in nursing research." *Journal of Advanced Nursing* **69**(12): 2622–2634. Available at: https://onlinelibrary.wiley.com/doi/full/10.1111/jan.12152.

Paley, J. (2008). "Spirituality and secularization: nursing and the sociology of religion." *Journal of Clinical Nursing* **17**: 175–186.

## John the trauma nurse

'"Trauma" is one of those words about whose meaning there is no consensus; or… [as] a word that everyone uses, yet it has no fixed meaning on which everyone agrees—and the constant usage of the word generates the illusion that everyone refers to the same phenomenon whenever the word "trauma" is mentioned' (http://psychoanalyzadnes.cz/2018/02/19/the-concept-of-trauma-in-lacanian-psychoanalysis/).

There are different conceptualisations of trauma at work in this narrative—and they are interacting. One is the name of the speciality 'trauma' medicine or nursing and the accompanying physical rupture that they deal with. The second is the shocking event or experience that John describes trauma nurses going through, often visual in nature, and the third is a psychoanalytic idea of trauma developed by Freud and, later, Lacan, where it is understood as an unavoidable part of human life. Birth itself is understood by some as a traumatic emergence into a foreign environment that the baby must experience. For others, the basic human trauma is the emergence into language—which is always somebody else's language—that the baby has to learn to use to articulate its needs. In psychoanalytic terms, trauma is that which cannot be symbolised and organised in language and which becomes, along with the unique way that the individual responds to it, a cornerstone of their identity, or subjectivity.

## Questions

- John talks about a colleague who appears to have the ability to 'compartmentalise' his response to trauma, to put it behind a closed door and 'move on'. Have you ever worked with a colleague who seemed to have this ability not to 'go under' after the most difficult events with patients? What do you think was going on?

- Do you think it is essential to 'routinise the traumatic' in nursing work? Can you think of examples you have experienced? What are the advantages and disadvantages? How far do you think this is an individual or a team-based characteristic?

## Reading

Lawler, D. (2009). "Test of Time: A Case Study in the Functioning of Social Systems as a Defence Against Anxiety: Rereading 50 Years On." *Clinical Child Psychology and Psychiatry* **14**(4): 523–530.

The Centre for Trauma, Healing and Growth at the Oxford Development Centre sets out its principles for working with people who have experienced trauma on its website at: www.oxforddevelopmentcentre. co.uk/stress-and-trauma/.

Tatano Beck, C. (2010). "Secondary Traumatic Stress in Nurses: A Systematic Review." *Archives of Psychiatric Nursing* **25**(1): 1–10.

## Miriam's story

When I started to read research into resilience undertaken with children, I noticed that one of the early differences of opinion concerned the significance of either the inner or outer world of the child. The innovative and controversial work of Sigmund Freud opened up an entirely new line of inquiry into the human psyche. Those who built on Freud's work were as likely to strongly disagree with him as to support his assertions. One of those who departed from some of Freud's main assumptions was John Bowlby (1907–1990), today mostly known for his attachment theory. A key difference between Freud and Bowlby was that the latter focused on observable events from a child's upbringing, whereas the former believed that it was the events that occurred in the imagination of the child that were the origin of psychic problems. Perhaps Bowlby was caught up in that typically Anglo-Saxon empiricism.[3] Freud and some of those who followed him would tend to believe that it is the meaning that events have for each individual that is of crucial importance, rather than some objective inventory of actions and events. Much research into resilience among nurses sees leaving the profession as evidence of a lack of resilience while staying 'at the bedside' shows that a nurse is resilient. Miriam's story makes it painfully clear that observation of an individual's actions tells us little about the possible trauma that they may be experiencing.

## Questions

- Thinking about nurses, or others, that you have known or worked alongside, do some appear to thrive on adversity (to use a popular phrase) while others seem to collapse?
- Do some seem to encounter more than their fair share of adversity—in its various forms?
- Thinking of traumatic events during your own nursing career, do you think you could have been prepared for them? In what ways?

---

3 See Critchley (2001) if you are interested in the philosophical debate between empiricism and rationalism, the latter generally associated with 'continental' philosophy. Perhaps the most recent manifestation of this fundamental difference of thinking is Brexit.

## Reading

Chambliss, D. F. (1996). *Beyond caring, hospitals, nurses and the social organization of ethics.* Chicago, Chicago University Press.

Evans, A. M., D. A. Pereira and J. M. Parker (2008). "Occupational distress in nursing: A psychoanalytic reading of the literature." *Nursing Philosophy* **9**: 195–204.

Smith, P. (1992). *The Emotional Labour of Nursing.* Basingstoke, Macmillan Education.

Traynor, M. and A. Evans (2014). "Slavery and jouissance: analysing complaints of suffering in UK and Australian nurses' talk about their work." *Nursing Philosophy* **15**(3): 192–200.

## An anonymous story

This story concerns an employee's troubled relationship with her employer. It combines fragments of an uncertain trauma, possibly to do with a clinical error and its aftermath, an account of an NMC hearing from the point of view of a 'charged' registrant, along with comments about whistle-blowing. The relationship between the 'incident' that is never fully described and the teller's various acts of apparent whistle-blowing is unclear.

## Questions

- The anonymous teller writes in a certain 'tone of voice', which is particularly apparent if you read some passages aloud. How would you describe this tone? What do you think accounts for it?
- If you have made, or have come close to making, a clinical error, how was this dealt with in the workplace? Was it dealt with in a satisfactory way?
- Have you ever worked with someone who had been or became a whistle-blower? How did you respond to them?
- The nurse at the heart of this story made the decision not to return to nursing work. What do you think about this?

## Reading

The NMC publishes guidance about what that organisation considers to be whistle-blowing: www.nmc.org.uk/standards/guidance/raising-concerns-guidance-for-nurses-and-midwives/whistleblowing/.

Researchers have looked into the effects of whistle-blowing on those who do so. See the following references:

Jackson, D., K. Peters, S. Andrew, M. Edenborough, E. Halcomb, L. Luck, Y. Salamonson and L. Wilkes (2010). "Understanding whistleblowing: qualitative insights from nurse whistleblowers." *Journal of Advanced Nursing* 66(10): 2194–2201.

McDonald, S. and K. Ahern (2002). "The professional consequences of whistleblowing by nurses." *Journal of Professional Nursing* 16(6): 313–321.

The notes of NMC hearings are available here: www.nmc.org.uk/concerns-nurses-midwives/hearings/.

## Yasmin, the nurse who was bullied and who bit back

A 2015 poll (www.tuc.org.uk/news/nearly-third-people-are-bullied-work-says-tuc) carried out by YouGov for the Trades Union Congress (TUC) found that:

TOURO COLLEGE LIBRARY

- nearly a third of people (29%) are bullied at work
- women (34%) are more likely to be victims of bullying than men (23%)
- the highest prevalence of workplace bullying is among 40- to 59-year-olds, where 34% of adults are affected
- in nearly three-quarters (72%) of cases the bullying is carried out by a manager
- more than one in three (36%) people leave their job as a result of bullying.

Another survey by the Chartered Institute of Personnel and Development found that the groups most likely to experience bullying and harassment are black and Asian employees, women and people with a disability. Nearly one-third (29%) of Asian employees or those from other ethnic groups reported having experienced some form of bullying or harassment, compared with 18% of white employees.

Bullying is a difficult subject to deal with because it is so emotive, as is evident in Yasmin's story and especially in her dream.

## Questions

- Have you ever felt bullied at work? Do any of the common features of bullying listed above apply to your situation? How did the situation end? Or is it still on-going? If the latter, what are your plans to resolve it?

## Reading

The UK government offers basic advice about workplace bullying and harassment here: www.gov.uk/workplace-bullying-and-harassment.

A list of web-based resources from a training organisation that focuses on mental health issues at work is here: www.in-equilibrium.co.uk/bullying-awareness-resources/.

Many trades unions and other organisations offer advice to anyone who feels they are being bullied at work. The TUC's resource is on their website (www.tuc.org.uk) on this page: www.tuc.org.uk/workplace-issues/health-and-safety/bullying/bullied-work-dont-suffer-silence. There is a guide for workplace representative's here: www.tuc.org.uk/resource/bullying-work-guidance-safety-representatives. Please look at these or other resources. In summary, the advice is: do not suffer alone; speak to the bully (if appropriate—sometimes just one instance of standing up to them can stop them); keep a diary or other record; get advice from a trade union representative or legal adviser and understand the character of what is happening.

Yasmin's disturbing dream raises the issue of the abuse of male power. If it has raised particular issues for you, Rape Crisis England and Wales offers emotional support, information and self-help tools at https://rapecrisis.org.uk/. The International Society for Traumatic Stress Studies offers resources and information about recovered memories of childhood trauma at www.istss.org/public-resources/what-is-childhood-trauma/remembering-childhood-trauma.aspx. The same website provides video stories from survivors of trauma, one of which also includes a description of troubling dreams: www.istss.org/public-resources/survivors-talk-about-trauma.aspx.

## Marta, the migrant nurse

The migration of nurses is not new. UK governments have recruited doctors, nurses and other health workers from overseas to work in UK health services since the 1930s. The creation of the

NHS in 1948 greatly increased the need for nurses and others. The first large-scale recruitment of nurses from the Caribbean took place in the 1950s (see Chapter 8). Although governments tightened immigration controls during the 1960s and 1970s, the increasing demand for overseas health workers continued. Discrimination around training and career opportunities of first-generation overseas health workers, however, has had negative consequences. Shortfalls in certain fields of nursing and medicine continue and are predicted to intensify because of an international shortage of health workers (Snow and Jones 2011).

Migration is politically sensitive. Fear about what were considered to be inadequately controlled levels of migration into the UK by EU citizens, particularly those from newly admitted Eastern European countries, was probably the single biggest factor that drove the UK public's vote to leave the European Union. After the Brexit vote in 2016, racist attacks on migrants in the UK rose (Dearden 2017). The UK government operates a list of shortage occupations into which employers are permitted to recruit workers from outside the UK. Nursing is currently on this list (http://workpermit.com/immigration/united-kingdom/uk-tier-2-shortage-occupation-list).

## Questions

- This chapter focuses on migration into the UK after World War II (1936–45) but the issues that Marta's story raises have not gone away. If you have moved to the UK—or any other country—for work, is there anything familiar about Marta's story?
- Marta appeared to be reluctant to speak about any experiences of prejudice but we know from other contemporary accounts that it was common for German immigrants to face discrimination and sometimes suspicion and hostility in the UK. Do you think that migrants today, whether nurses you work or study with or others, are more willing to speak about their negative experiences?
- Research shows discrimination against overseas-trained nurses as well as black and minority ethnic nurses in the NHS. What kinds of discrimination are there? Some 'microaggressions' are subtle—to observers, though not to those affected.[4]

## Reading

Smith P. A., H. Allan, L. W Henry, J. A Larsen, and M. M. Mackintosh (2006) "Valuing and Recognising the Talents of a Diverse Healthcare Workforce", *Report from the REOH Study: Researching Equal Opportunities for Overseas-trained Nurses and Other Healthcare Professionals.* European Institute of Health and Medical Sciences, University of Surrey, the Open University and the Royal College of Nursing.

Buchan, J. and J. Sochalski (2004). "The migration of nurses: Trends and policies." *Bulletin of World Health Organization* **82**(8): 587–594.

Allan, H., H. Cowie and P. Smith (2009). "Overseas nurses' experiences of discrimination: a case of racist bullying." *Journal of Nursing Management* **17**: 898–906.

---

4 Microaggression is a term used for brief and commonplace daily verbal, behavioural, or environmental indignities, whether intentional or unintentional, that communicate hostile, derogatory, or negative prejudicial slights and insults toward any marginalized group (Sue 2010).

# BIBLIOGRAPHY

Allan, H., H. Cowie and P. Smith (2009). "Overseas nurses' experiences of discrimination: a case of racist bullying." *Journal of Nursing Management* **17**: 898–906.

Allan, H., M. Traynor, D. Kelly and P. Smith (2016). Becoming a Nurse. *Understanding Sociology in Nursing*. London, Sage: 50–70.

Althusser, L. (1971). *For Marx*. London, Allen Lane.

Anthony, E. J. and B. J. Cohler, Eds. (1987). *The Invulnerable Child*. The Guildford Psychiatry Series. New York, The Guilford Press.

BBC One Web Team Blog. (2009, 12th October). "Margaret Haywood allowed to practice again." Retrieved 22nd January 2018, from www.bbc.co.uk/blogs/panorama/2009/10/margaret_haywood_allowed_to_pr.html.

Borges, J. L. (2000). Ragnarok. *Labyrinths: Selected stories and other writings*. London, Penguin Books.

Brennan, G. and R. McSherry (2007). "Exploring the transition and professional socialisation from health care assistant to student nurse." *Nurse Education in Practice* **7**(4): 206–214.

Buchan, J., A. Charlesworth, B. Gershlick and I. Seccombe (2017). *Rising pressure: the NHS workforce challenge: Workforce profile and trends of the NHS in England*. London, The Health Foundation.

Buchan, J. and J. Sochalski (2004). "The migration of nurses: Trends and policies." *Bulletin of World Health Organization* **82**(8): 587–594.

Buchanan, D., D. Denyer, J. Jaina, C. Kelliher, C. Moore, E. Parry and C. Pilbeam (2013). "How do they manage? A qualitative study of the realities of middle and front-line management work in health care." *Health Services and Delivery Research*, 1(4).

Burbules, N. and R. Berk. (1999). Critical Thinking and Critical Pedagogy: Relations, Differences, and Limits. In *Critical theories in education*. T. Popkewitz and L. Fendler (Eds.). New York, Routledge.

Butler, J. (2001). "Giving an Account of Oneself." *Diacritics* **31**(4): 22–40.

Cartwright, S. and C. L. Cooper (2007). "Hazards to health: The problem of workplace bullying." *The psychologist* 20(5): 284–287.

Chambliss, D. F. (1996). *Beyond caring, hospitals, nurses and the social organization of ethics*. Chicago, Chicago University Press.

Charlesworth, A. and S. Lafond (2017). "Shifting from undersupply to oversupply: Does NHS workforce planning need a paradigm shift?" *Economic Affairs* **37**(1): 36–52.

Chicago Women's Liberation Union. (1970). "Consciousness-Raising by The Women's Collective (Archive)." Retrieved 11th January 2018, from www.cwluherstory.org/classic-feminist-writings-articles/consciousness-raising.

Critchley, S. (2001). *Continental Philosophy. A very short introduction*. Oxford, Oxford University Press.

Davis, C. (1997) "Poetry about patients: Hearing the nurse's voice." *Journal of Medical Humanities* 18(2), 111–125.

Dearden, L. (2017, 17th October). "Hate-crime reports rise by almost a third in year as Home Office figures illustrate EU-referendum spike: Police figures also show huge rise in reports following terror attacks." *The Independent.*

Department of Health (2009) *Religion or Belief: a Practical Guide for the NHS.* Available at www. clatterbridgecc.nhs.uk/application/files/7214/3445/0178/ReligionorbeliefApracticalguideforthe NHS.pdf.

Dolan, G., E. Strodl and E. Hamernik (2012). "Why renal nurses cope so well with their workplace stressors." *Journal of Renal Care* **38**(4): 222–232.

Dyer, J. G. and T. McGuinness (1996). "Resilience: analysis of the concept." *Archives of Psychiatric Nursing* 10(5): 276–282.

Dyson, S. (2018). *Critical Pedagogy in Nursing.* Basingstoke, Palgrave Macmillan.

Earvolino-Ramirez, M. (2007). "Resilience: a concept analysis." *Nursing Forum* **42**(2): 73–82.

East, L., D. Jackson, L. O'Brien and K. Peters (2010). "Storytelling: an approach that can help to develop resilience." *Nurse Researcher* **17**(3): 17–25.

Eliot, T. S. (1919). "Tradition and the Individual Talent." *The Egoist.* Available at http://tseliot.com/ essays/tradition-and-the-individual-talent.

Empey, D. (2004). "Editorial: Suspension of doctors." *BMJ* **328**:: 181–182.

Fagan, J. (2004). *Suspension failure in the NHS: Report for Brian Jenkins MP, member of the Public Accounts Committee.*

Evans, A. M., D. A. Pereira and J. M. Parker (2008). "Occupational distress in nursing: A psychoanalytic reading of the literature." *Nursing Philosophy* 9: 195–204.

Frank, A. (2010). *Letting Stories Breathe: a socio-narratology.* Chicago, University of Chicago Press.

Freidson, E. (1970). *The Profession of Medicine: a study of the sociology of applied knowledge.* Chicago, University of Chicago Press.

Freire, P. (1970). *Pedagogy of the oppressed.* New York, Herder and Herder.

Freud, S. (1990). *Case Histories I: 'Dora' and 'Little Hans' (The Penguin Freud Library, Vol. 8).* London, Penguin.

Freud, S. (2001). *Totem and Taboo: some points of agreement between the mental lives of savages and neurotics.* Abingdon, Routledge.

Friborg, O., O. Hjemdal, J. H. Rosenvinge and M. Martinussen (2003). "A new rating scale for adult resilience: what are the central protective resources behind healthy adjustment?" *International Journal of Methods in Psychiatric Research* **12**(2): 65–76.

Henry, W. L. (2012). "Reggae, Rasta and the Role of the Deejay in the Black British Experience." *Contemporary British History* **26**(3): 355–373.

Holoyda, B. and W. Newman (2016). "Between Belief and Delusion: Cult Members and the Insanity Plea." *Journal of the American Academy of Psychiatry and the Law* **44**(1): 53–62.

House of Commons Committee of Public Accounts (2016). *Managing the Supply of NHS Clinical Staff in England.* London, House of Commons.

Howkins, E. J. and A. Ewens (1999). "How students experience professional socialisation." *International Journal of Nursing Studies* **36**(1): 41–49.

Iyassu, R., S. Jolley, P. Bebbington, G. Dunn, R. Emsley, D. Freeman, D. Fowler, A. Hardy, H. Waller, E. Kuipers and P. Garety (2014). "Psychological characteristics of religious delusions." *Social Psychiatry and Psychiatric Epidemiology* 49(7): 1051–1061.

Jack, K. (2015) "The use of poetry writing in nurse education: An evaluation." *Nurse Education Today* 35(9), e7–e10.

Jackson, D., A. Fau-Firtko and M. Edenborough (2007). "Personal resilience as a strategy for surviving and thriving in the face of workplace adversity: a literature review." *Journal of Advanced Nursing* 60(1): 1–9.

Jackson, D., K. Peters, S. Andrew, M. Edenborough, E. Halcomb, L. Luck, Y. Salamonson and L. Wilkes (2010). "Understanding whistleblowing: qualitative insights from nurse whistleblowers." *Journal of Advanced Nursing* 66(10): 2194–2201.

Koen, M. P., C. van Eeden and M. P. Wissing (2011). "The prevalence of resilience in a group of professional nurses." *Health SA Gesondheid* **16**(1): 1–11.

Labov, W., Ed. (1972). *Language in the inner city: Studies in the Black English vernacular.* Philadelphia, University of Pennsylvania Press.

Larrabee, J. H., Y. Wu, C. A. Persily, P. S. Simoni, P. A. Johnston, T. L. Marcischak, C. L. Mott and S. D. Gladden (2010). "Influence of stress resiliency on RN job satisfaction and intent to stay." *Western Journal of Nursing Research* **32**(1): 81–102.

Lawler, D. (2009). "Test of Time: A Case Study in the Functioning of Social Systems as a Defence Against Anxiety: Rereading 50 Years On." *Clinical Child Psychology and Psychiatry* **14**(4): 523–530.

Luthar, S. S. and D. Cicchetti (2000). "The construct of resilience: Implications for interventions and social policies." *Development and Psychopathology* **12**(4): 857–885.

Maben, J., S. Latter and J. M. Clark (2007). "The sustainability of ideals, values and the nursing mandate: evidence from a longitudinal qualitative study." *Nursing Inquiry* **14**(2): 99–113.

Mackintosh, C. (2006). "Caring: The socialisation of pre-registration student nurses: A longitudinal qualitative descriptive study." *International Journal of Nursing Studies* **43**(8): 953–962.

Masten, A. S. and J. Obradović (2006). "Competence and Resilience in Development." *Annals of the New York Academy of Sciences* **1094**(1): 13–27.

Matos, P. S., L. A. Neushotz, M. T. Q. Griffin and J. J. Fitzpatrick (2010). "An exploratory study of resilience and job satisfaction among psychiatric nurses working in inpatient units." *International Journal of Mental Health Nursing* **19**(5): 307–312.

McAdams, D. P. and E. Manczak (2015). Personality and the Life Story. In *APA Handbook of Personality and Social Psychology.* M. Mikulincer and P. R. Shaver (Eds.). Washington, American Psychological Association.

McDonald, S. and K. Ahern (2002). "The professional consequences of whistleblowing by nurses." *Journal of Professional Nursing* **16**(6): 313–321.

Mealer, M., J. Jones, J. Newman, K. K. McFann, B. Rothbaum and M. Moss (2012). "The presence of resilience is associated with a healthier psychological profile in intensive care unit (ICU) nurses: Results of a national survey." *International Journal of Nursing Studies* **49**(3): 292–299.

Melia, K. M. (1987). *Learning and Working: The Occupational Socialization of Nurses.* London, Tavistock.

Memmi, A. ([1957] 1991). *The Colonizer and the Colonized.* Boston, Beacon Press.

National Audit Office (2016). *Managing the Supply of NHS Clinical staff in England.* London, NAO.

Neocleous, M. (2013). "Resisting resilience." *Radical Philosophy* **178**: 6.

NHS Digital. (2016, November). "NHS Workforce Statistics – August 2016, Provisional statistics." Retrieved 11th March 2017, from http://content.digital.nhs.uk/searchcatalogue?productid=23451&topics=0%2fWorkforce&sort=Relevance&size=10&page=1 – top.

O'Driscoll, M. F., H. T. Allan and P. A. Smith (2010). "Still looking for leadership – Who is responsible for student nurses' learning in practice?" *Nurse education today* **30**(3): 212–217.

O'Malley, P. (2009). Responsibilization. In *The Sage Dictionary of Policing.* A. Wakefield and J. Fleming (Eds.). London, Sage: 276–277.

Page, B. (2016, 26th April). "No matter what Jeremy Hunt does, the statistics show that we will always trust a doctor over a government minister." *The Independent.*

Paley, J. (2008). "Spirituality and secularization: nursing and the sociology of religion." *Journal of Clinical Nursing* **17**: 175–186.

Pirsig, R., M (1983). *Zen and the Art of Motorcycle Maintenance: An inquiry into Values.* London, Corgi Books.

Pittman, P., L. H. Aiken and J. Buchan (2007). "International Migration of Nurses: Introduction." *Health Services Research* **42**(3 Pt 2): 1275–1280.

Public Records Office (1949). *Scheme for Training German Girls as State Registered Nurses in Great Britain.* London, Ministry of Labour: **8/1305**.

Randall, W., C. Baldwin, S. McKenzie-Mohr, E. McKim and D. Furlong (2015). "Narrative and resilience: A comparative analysis of how older adults story their lives." *Journal of Aging Studies* **34**: 155–161.

Reinert, K. G. and H. G. Koenig (2013). "Re-examining definitions of spirituality in nursing research." *Journal of Advanced Nursing* **69**(12): 2622–2634. Available at https://onlinelibrary.wiley.com/doi/full/10.1111/jan.12152.

Riessman, C. K. (1993). *Narrative Analysis*. Newbury Park, CA, Sage.

Rutter, M. (1985). "Resilience in the Face of Adversity: Protective Factors and Resistance to Psychiatric Disorder." *British Journal of Psychiatry* **147**: 598–611.

Seccombe, I., G. Smith, J. Buchan and J. Ball (1997). ENROLLED NURSES: a study for the UKCC. Brighton, Institute for Employment Studies.

Simms, A. (2012). "Religious Delusions." Retrieved 8th August 2018, from www.rcpsych.ac.uk/docs/default-source/members/sigs/spirituality-spsig/is-faith-delusion-andrew-sims-editedx.pdf?sfvrsn=59a019c0_2.

Smith, P. (1992). *The Emotional Labour of Nursing*. Basingstoke, Macmillan Education.

Snow, S. and E. Jones. (2011, March). "Immigration and the National Health Service: putting history to the forefront." *Policy Papers*. Retrieved 28th September 2018, from www.historyandpolicy.org/policy-papers/papers/immigration-and-the-national-health-service-putting-history-to-the-forefron.

Speare, J. and Henshall, A. (2014) "'Did anyone think the trees were students?' Using poetry as a tool for critical reflection." *Reflective Practice: International and Multidisciplinary Perspectives.* 15(6), 1–14.

Sue, D. W. (2010). *Microaggressions in Everyday Life: Race, Gender, and Sexual Orientation*. New Jersey, Wiley.

Tatano Beck, C. (2010). "Secondary Traumatic Stress in Nurses: A Systematic Review." *Archives of Psychiatric Nursing* **25**(1): 1–10.

Tevendale, F. and D. Armstrong (2015). "Using patient storytelling in nurse education." *Nursing Times* **111**(6): 15–17.

Traynor, M. (2013). *Nursing in Context: policy politics profession*. Basingstoke, Palgrave.

Traynor, M. (2017). *Critical Resilience for Nurses: an evidence-based Guide to survival and Change in the Modern NHS*. Abingdon, Routledge.

Traynor, M. and A. Evans (2014). "Slavery and jouissance: analysing complaints of suffering in UK and Australian nurses' talk about their work." *Nursing Philosophy* **15**(3): 192–200.

Weber-Newth, I. and J.-D. Steinert (2006). *German Migrants in Post-War Britain: An Enemy Embrace*. Oxford, Routledge.

Williams, R. and P. Hazell (2011). "Austerity, poverty, resilience, and the future of mental health services for children and adolescents." *Current Opinion in Psychiatry* 24(4): 263–266.

Winders, S. (2014). "From extraordinary invulnerability to ordinary magic: A literature review of resilience." *Journal of European Psychology Students* 5(1): 3–9.

Yansori, A. (2018, 19th February). "The Concept of Trauma in Lacanian Psychoanalysis." Retrieved 29th November 2018, from http://psychoanalyzadnes.cz/2018/02/19/the-concept-of-trauma-in-lacanian-psychoanalysis/.

Zander, M., A. Hutton and L. King (2010). "Coping and resilience factors in pediatric oncology nurses." *Journal of Pediatric Oncology Nursing* **27**(2): 94–108.

# INDEX

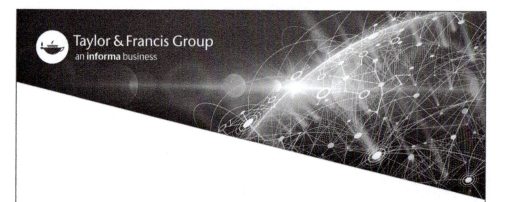

Taylor & Francis Group
an **informa** business

# Taylor & Francis eBooks

www.taylorfrancis.com

A single destination for eBooks from Taylor & Francis with increased functionality and an improved user experience to meet the needs of our customers.

90,000+ eBooks of award-winning academic content in Humanities, Social Science, Science, Technology, Engineering, and Medical written by a global network of editors and authors.

## TAYLOR & FRANCIS EBOOKS OFFERS:

A streamlined experience for our library customers

A single point of discovery for all of our eBook content

Improved search and discovery of content at both book and chapter level

## REQUEST A FREE TRIAL
support@taylorfrancis.com

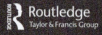
Routledge
Taylor & Francis Group

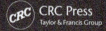
CRC Press
Taylor & Francis Group